WHAT YOU NEED TO KNOW ABOUT RITALIN

- How do I know if I have ADHD?
- Is ADHD inherited?
- Will my child outgrow ADHD?
- Can Ritalin stunt her growth?
- Should I worry about my teenager abusing Ritalin?
- What rights does my ADHD child have in school?
- Can Ritalin make me smarter?
- How will I feel if I take Ritalin?
- Can Ritalin cause Tourette's syndrome?
- Are other drugs as good . . . or better?

GET ANSWERS YOU CAN TRUST,
IN LANGUAGE YOU CAN UNDERSTAND

WHAT YOU NEED TO KNOW ABOUT RITALIN

James Shaya, M.D., James Windell,
and Holly Shreve Gilbert

New York   Toronto   London   Sydney   Auckland

WHAT YOU NEED TO KNOW ABOUT RITALIN

A Bantam Book / March 1999

Reprinted with permission from the Diagnostic and Statistical Manual of Mental Disorders, Fourth Edition. Copyright 1994 American Psychiatric Association.

Copyright © 1997 Multi-Health Systems Inc., 908 Niagara Falls Blvd., North Tonawanda, New York, 14120-2060, (800) 456-3003. Reproduced by permission.

ISBN 0-553-57552-X

Published simultaneously in the United States and Canada

Bantam Books are published by Bantam Books, a division of Random
House, Inc. Its trademark, consisting of the words "Bantam Books" and
the portrayal of a rooster, is Registered in U.S. Patent and Trademark
Office and in other countries. Marca Registrada. Bantam Books, 1540
Broadway, New York, New York 10036.

PRINTED IN THE UNITED STATES OF AMERICA

OPM   10   9   8   7   6   5   4   3   2   1

To

Ellen, Isabella, and Matthew,

and Garry and Jackson

CONTENTS

ACKNOWLEDGMENTS

*T*he authors would like to thank the many professionals who shared their time and expertise, especially:

Dr. Robert Resnick, Dr. James Swanson, Dr. Martin Baren, Dr. Arthur Robin, Dr. Marcia Rappley, Dr. Michael Gordon, Dr. Howard Schubner, Michael Merz, and Tom Harwood.

Without the gracious cooperation of dozens of ADHD patients, parents, and members of CHADD, this book would not have been possible.

PUBLISHER'S NOTE

WHAT YOU NEED TO KNOW ABOUT RITALIN

CHAPTER ONE

What Is Ritalin?

Millions of American children and adults begin each day by swallowing a central nervous system stimulant called Ritalin.

In the past twenty years, the little blue or yellow pill has become the drug of choice in treating attention deficit hyperactivity disorder (ADHD), the most frequently diagnosed behavioral disorder in children and one of the fastest-growing diagnoses of adults in the United States.[1]

Experts estimate that as many as 12.5 million Americans suffer from various degrees of this condition, characterized by three primary symptoms of inattentiveness, hyperactivity, and impulsivity.[2]

Although you may have just started hearing about ADHD during the past ten years, the only thing remotely new about it is its name. The symptoms have been observed for at least half a century. During most of that time, however, they were misinterpreted and mislabeled. In fact, as recently as a generation ago, school-age children who suffered from ADHD were often written off as disciplinary problems. They were punished instead of helped.

"I spent a lot more time standing in the corner than I did sitting at my desk," says "Frank Lee." (Most of the names in the case studies in this book are pseudonyms, which will be denoted by placing quotation marks around the name the first time it is mentioned.) The 52-year-old salesman says he still flinches when he thinks about his miserable school years. He was diagnosed with ADHD when he was 45 and started taking Ritalin soon after.

Now that Frank, like a lot of us, knows better, he's making sure the same thing doesn't happen to his son, who also has ADHD.

Because we understand ADHD better today, we can assess it and treat it more effectively. Ritalin is often the cornerstone of a successful treatment program; as many as 90 percent of children diagnosed with ADHD will be prescribed Ritalin in the course of their treatment.[3]

Because of Ritalin's effectiveness, use of the drug is at an all-time high. Prescriptions increased 450 percent from 1991 to 1995, climbing from a nationwide consumption of 4,000 pounds to 18,000 pounds annually, according to the Drug Enforcement Administration (DEA).[4]

Even before Ritalin use increased so dramatically, the drug was making headlines. You may have seen it portrayed in the media as a dangerous drug. Some news stories have claimed that Ritalin can cause psychotic behavior. For example, a 1987 story in the *Detroit News* explained, "The manufacturer of Ritalin warns in its packaging materials that 'chronically abusive use can lead to marked tolerance and psychic dependence with varying degrees of abnormal behavior.' It also cautions that 'careful supervision is required during drug withdrawal, since severe depression as well as the effects of chronic overactivity can be unmasked.' "[5]

The quotation, which is also cited by many Ritalin opponents, is accurate, but it was used out of context. In the *Physicians' Desk Reference* the boxed warning actually begins with this paragraph:

> Ritalin should be given cautiously to emotionally unstable patients, such as those with a history of drug dependence or alcoholism, because such patients may increase dosage on their own initiative.

Also missing from the opponents' version of the quote is this sentence: "Frank psychotic episodes can occur, especially with parenteral [intravenous] abuse."

These complete sentences make it obvious that the warning is intended for unstable or emotionally disturbed patients, not for hyperactive seven-year-olds who are otherwise mentally and physically sound. So yes, Ritalin can, in rare instances, be dangerous. But so can many drugs when given to patients with psychotic tendencies, when given in very high doses, or when given to patients who are far too young to tolerate them.[6]

You've probably heard Ritalin compared to cocaine. It's true that the two drugs are chemically similar in nature;[7] both are short-acting stimulants derived synthetically from amphetamine. But unlike cocaine, Ritalin has beneficial medicinal value. For instance, besides its popular use as an ADHD remedy, it's also employed to treat the sleep disorder narcolepsy.

Like cocaine, Ritalin has an abuse potential. But says Dr. Russell Barkley, a professor of psychiatry and neurology at the University of Massachusetts Medical Center and the author of *Attention Deficit Hyperactivity Disorder: A Handbook for Diagnosis and Treatment*, "For this drug to be potentially addictive, it has to be crushed and inhaled nasally, or injected, and that has to be done repeatedly." Dr. Barkley, who runs an ADHD clinic at the University of Massachusetts, says, "When taken orally, as prescribed, there is no risk of addiction."[8]

According to the Harvard Medical School's *Harvard Mental Health Letter*, "little danger of drug abuse or addiction" is associated with Ritalin because unlike recreational drugs, it doesn't cause children and adults with ADHD to "feel euphoria or develop tolerance or craving."[9] The newsletter goes on to report that individuals with ADHD may become dependent on Ritalin or other stimulant medications only in the same sense that a person with diabetes is dependent on insulin.

Ritalin shouldn't be prescribed to people with a history of drug dependence or alcoholism, since their tolerances or cravings are unpredictable.[10]

Probably the most frightening things you've heard lately about Ritalin are stories of young people snorting or injecting the drug. If you've watched prime-time TV, you've probably also seen reports about individuals and groups trafficking in Ritalin. The DEA confirms that such stories are true.[11] But again, missing are the stories of the millions of children and untold numbers of adults who are presently undergoing successful, legitimate Ritalin therapy.[12] More than two-thirds of them will improve with no serious side effects.[13]

What is Ritalin, Exactly?

Ritalin, the brand name for the drug methylphenidate, is a short-acting stimulant medication manufactured by Novartis (formerly Ciba–Geigy Pharmaceuticals). It's dispensed in 5, 10, and 20 milligram tablets that usually begin to work within a half hour after ingestion. Effectiveness typically begins to dwindle within four hours, as the drug clears from the body, making it necessary to take second and sometimes third doses during the day.[14]

Because more than one dose is generally required

each day, Ritalin is often dispensed in school. The educational community has been grappling with this issue and attempting to provide solutions to the problems that Ritalin dispensing can present. Leaving a child's medication program in the hands of a teacher or school secretary, for example, may be unsettling to the parents. You can find out more about how to deal with these situations in Chapter 7.

Sustained-release (SR) Ritalin can provide a viable alternative to the school dilemma. This longer-acting form of the pill—which has helped to increase Ritalin's popularity—delivers 10 milligrams immediately and another 10 milligrams about four hours later. Although the SR form is more practical, many children and adults find it's not quite as effective as the short-acting pill.[15]

Most major health insurance companies recognize ADHD as a valid psychological diagnosis and offer some form of reimbursement for Ritalin. The pills themselves are relatively inexpensive, costing from 25 to 50 cents each, depending on where they are dispensed. There is a generic form of Ritalin called methylphenidate hydrochloride, which is less expensive than the brand-name drug. Some people report a noticeable difference in the way the generic and brand name drugs affect them—after taking the brand-name drug, for example, the equivalent generic may seem less effective. This is probably because differences in their potencies may be discernible. As Dr. Ruth Robin of the Attention Deficit Center in Southfield, Michigan, explains, "Generic drugs only have to be 75 percent as effective [as brand names]. If you start with generic, stay with generic."[16]

To discourage abuse of Ritalin, the DEA has designated it as a "Schedule II controlled substance." This means it's subject to rigid yearly manufacturing quotas. As a consequence, supply, particularly in the past several years, hasn't always kept up with the growing demand.[17]

Because of federal restrictions on controlled drugs, pharmacists scrutinize requests for Ritalin. Handwritten prescriptions are required and must be filled within five days of the physician's request. Refills are not an option.

Therefore it's in your best interest to make appointments for follow-up doctor visits in a timely fashion. Don't wait until your prescription has almost run out before trying to fit in a visit—if the doctor can't see you, or if there are any snags at the pharmacy, your prescription may lapse.

The Stimulant Paradox

The very idea of using a stimulant to remedy hyperactivity and impulsivity seems to fly in the face of common sense. But doctors discovered a long time ago that drugs like Ritalin actually work on the parts of the brain involved in attention. Ritalin helps people sort and prioritize the constant stream of information that bombards them every second. In effect, Ritalin allows the brain to slow down, filter extraneous information, and focus on the matter at hand.

Stimulants were first used to treat behavior problems in the late 1930s, when benzedrine was administered to a group of difficult children who had been confined to an inpatient ward. Their conduct improved, and so did their school performance. Subsequent studies produced similar results, and in the meantime, in the mid-1950s, Ritalin entered the pharmaceutical stimulant market. The drug crept along in popularity until the late 1970s, when it pushed other ADHD treatments, such as diets and vitamins, into obscurity.[18] Although some still attempt to treat this disorder with diet and holistic medicine, research since the early 1970s continues to show no conclusive proof that such approaches work. (Alternative therapies are discussed in Chapters 6 and 9.)

What Ritalin Can Do

Ritalin has become a popular treatment for ADHD simply because it works. Study after study has demonstrated that Ritalin may effect real, measurable short-term improvement in children's behavior, in their schoolwork, and in their social relationships. To cite just a few of them:

• A 1992 study compared ADHD boys who were taking Ritalin with ADHD children who were not being treated with any medication. The children who took medication had higher academic self-esteem than the nonmedicated children.[19]

• In 1988 Russell Barkley evaluated the effects of Ritalin on young children's relationships with their mothers. He found that a high dose of methylphenidate significantly improved the children's willingness to obey their mothers.[20]

• Another study investigated the effects of Ritalin on the academic efforts and abilities of sixteen children diagnosed with ADHD. On a number of cognitive, academic, and behavioral measures, a majority of them showed improvements with increased accuracy, output, and efficiency.[21]

The medical literature contains dozens of studies showing similar findings. More research has been conducted on the effects of stimulant medications on children with ADHD than on *any* other treatment method for *any* childhood behavioral disorder.[22]

The most compelling testimonials to the effectiveness of Ritalin come from ADHD sufferers themselves. Before she was diagnosed with ADHD, "Anna Alden" was miserable in school. She found it impossible to stay in her seat or pay attention to her teacher. As a result, her grades were poor, and her attitude, not surprisingly, was completely negative. The worst part was that she suffered alone—she had no friends.

Now nine, the pigtailed third-grader tells stories about pajama parties and good grades.

"Tim Gabriel" says when he was Anna's age, he didn't have friends either. "You know the creepy kid in the class—well, that was me," he says. As a third-grader, he was a social outcast. His teachers were constantly reprimanding him for not paying attention, and his classmates totally ignored him. For Tim, lunch hour and recess were like solitary confinement.

But at 18, Tim is captain of his high school swim team and a National Merit Scholar. He takes Ritalin every day and believes he will continue it for the rest of his life. "Of course I'd like to kick the Ritalin," he says, "but my ADHD is severe."

Medical experts used to believe that people like Anna and Tim would eventually outgrow their ADHD. "Researchers once believed that the inattention, impulsiveness and hyperactivity of ADHD faded with the onset of adolescence," write Dr. Andrew Adesman and Dr. Esther H. Wender in *Contemporary Pediatrics*. "Although the gross motor hyperactivity does generally diminish, many hyperkinetic children continue to experience problems with fine motor coordination, restlessness, fidgetiness, inattentiveness, and distractibility into adolescence and adulthood."[23]

Increasingly, doctors and psychologists are diagnosing ADHD in adults and achieving dramatic results with Ritalin treatment. "Susan Phillips," for example, mother of two, has a hard time imagining how she lived so many years with ADHD and without Ritalin. She says she was a "chronically frustrated child" who had to work twice as hard as her friends just to do half as well.

At 35 she was diagnosed with ADHD, and at 36, she says, she's now hitting her stride. She's finally in college and thrilled not only to be doing well but to "comprehend what I'm doing."

Taking Ritalin isn't necessarily a lifelong commitment. Sometimes the drug enables people to focus to such a degree that they are able to develop the coping skills necessary to manage the disorder without medication. In Chapter 10 we'll discuss the behavior modification therapies useful in developing these skills.

What Ritalin Can't Do

RITALIN CAN'T MAKE YOU OR YOUR CHILD SMARTER.

Although a 1993 study indicated that for both children and adults, the use of Ritalin improved school performance, no drug has the capacity to raise IQ. When Ritalin is prescribed appropriately, it enhances the ability to learn by improving concentration, short-term memory, vigilance, impulse control, and fine motor skills. ADHD sufferers who take the drug don't get smarter, they just get more done.

RITALIN CAN'T CURE ADHD.

Nothing can cure ADHD. This disorder is caused by an imbalance in the brain's chemistry. Once a dose of Ritalin wears off, the brain chemicals return to their prior levels. Ritalin corrects the symptoms of ADHD, but only on a temporary basis.

RITALIN CAN'T BE USED TO DIAGNOSE ADHD.

A positive response to Ritalin doesn't establish the existence of ADHD. For some ADHD sufferers, Ritalin therapy simply doesn't work. And in rare cases the drug can actually mask indications of related disorders, such as learning disabilities and depression. An accurate diagnosis can be confirmed only by a series of assessments and evaluations performed by medical, psychological, and educational experts (as described in Chapter 4).

Ritalin's Side Effects

Although Ritalin has provided a huge breakthrough in the treatment of ADHD, some children and adults do experience certain side effects. According to Dr. Robert Findling, assistant professor of pediatrics and psychiatry at Case Western Reserve University in

Cleveland, "about 70 percent of people on Ritalin handle it well."[24]

These side effects can range from physical complaints, such as headaches, appetite suppression, and stomachaches, to psychological disturbances, such as sleep difficulties, tearfulness, and irritability. Usually these problems are mild and can be alleviated by adjusting the dosage schedule and modifying eating habits. For example, some children aren't hungry after taking their second dose of Ritalin, and because they don't eat, their stomachs hurt. Eating first, then taking the medicine, is a simple way to alleviate this problem. At any rate it's important to report any side effects to your doctor immediately. Sometimes all that's needed is a simple adjustment in dosage.

Questions of dosage and side effects are addressed more fully in Chapter 7.

Not a Magic Pill

As with most medical disorders, the follow-up care of ADHD is much more difficult than the diagnosis. Medication is never the sole answer to solving its many complexities.

Ritalin can be a strong foundation for therapy, but it is hardly the sole support. Treatment for ADHD must involve educational accommodations, academic tutoring, family therapy, and counseling (as described in Chapters 10 and 12). Each of these components requires more dedication than merely taking a pill two or three times a day.

The bottom line is that *you* are the most important part of any ADHD treatment program, whether it's your own or your child's. No pill is magic. And no pill, no matter how safe or effective, should be left to work entirely on its own.

CHAPTER TWO

What Is ADHD?

*A*ttention deficit hyperactivity disorder is troubling, it's misunderstood, and it's complex. But one adjective is probably used to describe ADHD more frequently than any other: frustrating.

Because of its vague symptoms and its complicated diagnostic process, ADHD is frustrating for physicians and psychologists alike. Because they often have to live with an emotionally volatile and often unresponsive child or adult, the disorder is also frustrating for family members and friends. And because one single case of it can disrupt an entire classroom, it's frustrating for teachers.

Mostly, though, ADHD is frustrating for the children or adults who have it—because they are almost always intelligent and capable, yet find it impossible to perform to their optimal level.

The causes of all these frustrations are ADHD's three primary symptoms—inattentiveness, hyperactivity, and impulsivity.

In toddlers and preschoolers various extremes of these symptoms are tolerable, even expected. But a kindergartner or first-grader who can't pay attention, follow directions, or sit still is a different story. In school-age children and adults, these behaviors interfere in learning processes and the development of social skills. Failures become chronic, depleting not only ambition but self-esteem.

Incidence of ADHD

A leading cause of school failure and underachievement, ADHD is thought to afflict as many as 10 percent of American children.[1] Skeptics often balk at this figure. Yet reliable research reported in professional journals has made estimates that range to up to 21 percent of school-age children.

These figures raise the question: Why do so many children today appear to have ADHD when past generations didn't seem to be afflicted by it? Russell Barkley has said that although the actual incidence of ADHD may not be on the rise, its detection may be increasing.[2]

The simple truth is that ADHD has been around

for years, but it was never as clearly understood as it is now. In the 1940s and 1950s, for example, children with ADHD were thought to be mentally retarded or brain damaged.[3] In the 1960s and 1970s, the symptoms of ADHD were classified as "minimal brain dysfunction."[4] Now doctors, psychologists, and educators have a clearer picture of what ADHD involves, recognize it more often, and treat it successfully.

Many adults are being assessed and treated, too.

Experts used to believe that ADHD symptoms disappeared during adolescence due to developmental or hormonal changes. In recent years, however, follow-up studies have demonstrated that 30 to 70 percent of children with ADHD symptoms continue to exhibit them throughout adolescence and adulthood.[5] Because of the phenomenal amount of publicity generated about ADHD during the past ten or fifteen years, more people know about it today. A lot of grown-ups are finally discovering they've been dealing with it for years.

While some experts contend that our society is on ADHD-information overload and it's become trendy and overdiagnosed, many children will still never be diagnosed or treated. Most of them are girls, despite the fact that three times as many boys are estimated to have ADHD.[6] Girls, more often than boys, have ADD—ADHD without hyperactivity—and the absence of that hallmark symptom often leads diagnosticians astray.[7] Then, too, assessment and treatment tend to seem more urgent when disruptive physical behavior is involved. The first-grade boy who jumps around the room and takes swipes at his little friends presents a pressing problem. The little girl who daydreams, in comparison, seems harmless enough.

To others, perhaps. But not to herself.

Effects of ADHD

If you're the parent of an ADHD child, you probably had a gut feeling that something wasn't quite right. You knew, for instance, that your rambunctious five-year-old had a lot of "spirit," but why couldn't he ever wait his turn in line? And why, even when he got in line, couldn't he remember what he was supposed to be doing there? Family and friends may have fed you the "boys will be boys" line. Even your doctor may have told you that there was nothing to worry about—yet.

It was probably a teacher who finally confirmed your suspicions. Being overwhelmed with school is one thing, but bouncing off the walls during reading lessons just doesn't cut it.

As soon as he got into school, "Eric Spencer's" problems started surfacing. At parent-teacher conferences his mom and dad heard comments like "Eric is a nice boy, but he has problems focusing and he just can't sit still." Like other ADHD children, Eric had a short attention span and couldn't keep his mind focused on his classroom tasks. "Eric doesn't pay attention," his third-grade teacher wrote on his report card, "and I know if he did, he would excel at all subjects."

Despite remaining undiagnosed and untreated for several more years, Eric muddled through.

Many ADHD children aren't so fortunate. The learning impairments imposed by their symptoms often drag them down and put them at greater risk of being held back in class. And the child who suffers scholastically ultimately endures a variety of social and emotional disturbances as well, which can escalate into problems that go far beyond the scope of ADHD and are far more challenging to treat.

If you're dealing with ADHD as an adult, you're probably facing a different set of struggles related to your restlessness, your distractibility, your mood swings, or your short temper. You know from experience that each of these behaviors can have a profound effect on your life.

What ADHD Is Not

Most professionals have difficulty providing a clear-cut definition of ADHD. There are no blood tests for diagnosing it, and it isn't an ailment, like measles or the flu, with clear physical signs. But they do agree on certain things that ADHD is *not*.

• ADHD is not the result of an accident, a psychological or physical trauma, or drug addiction. It is an inherent genetic disorder of brain dysfunction. It is part of the person's physical makeup and cannot be permanently corrected.

• Despite reports to the contrary, ADHD is not a result of radiation, TV, or the like. Nor is ADHD caused by allergies, sugar, food, or poor parenting. But, allergies, sugar—such as the sugar found in sweets, soda pop, and desserts—preservatives in food, and inconsistent parenting can exaggerate the symptoms of ADHD or even produce conditions resembling this disorder.[8]

• ADHD is not an indicator of low intelligence. Affected children may score lower than average on standardized intelligence tests because of the tests' bias toward good concentration skills. But the majority of people with ADHD are of average or above-average intelligence.[9]

Each of these issues is explained in more detail in Chapter 3.

What ADHD Is

The loosest definition of ADHD is "a syndrome characterized by the inability to filter information." Every waking moment of every day, the brain is being bombarded with information. At this moment you might feel the smooth cover of this book, hear a noise outside, and smell something in the air, yet you are able to concentrate only on the words on this page. People with ADHD, however, just don't have this ability to prioritize information into what is important and what is not. Therefore they allow all this extraneous information to interfere with their concentration on the task at hand. It may take them several minutes or even hours to finish reading this one page.

How Does ADHD Feel?

One person has said that having ADHD is like being in a dark room where objects are scattered around to trip you. You don't get a flashlight, but everyone else does. You trip around the room, bumping into things, until you finally learn the layout. Then someone moves you to a new room, and the process starts over.

Tim Gabriel compares it to watching television. "Imagine you're watching twelve channels all at once," he says, "and you've lost your remote control."

Symptoms of ADHD

No two people exhibit ADHD in exactly the same way. It has many potential symptoms, and people show just as many extremes of them. Complicating the issue is the fact that many of these symptoms bear striking similarities to such closely related disorders as anxiety and depression.

There are, however, three symptoms that, when exhibited for six months or more, strongly suggest the possibility of ADHD.[10]

INATTENTIVENESS

For children and adults with ADHD, paying attention is next to impossible.

Inattentiveness in a child presents a double frustration—one for the child and one for the parent. If your child has ADHD, you're probably used to repeating instructions dozens of times. And you no doubt hate the thought of homework because night after night it turns into an endurance test—of your patience.

"Maria Gallardo," who was ten before her ADHD was diagnosed, found it agonizing to do homework. Although she had good intentions, the slightest noise would distract her from her work, and her attention would wander away from her math problems, her science projects, and her reading. "It was a nightmare," says her father, "Joe." "I just felt like we were nagging her all the time, but if we didn't, she would never see a passing grade."

Academic performance is often compromised in children with ADHD, although it's not a specific learning disability. One way of looking at it is that the ADHD child is not unable to learn; he or she is simply "unavailable" to learn.

The problem, as Russell Barkley has pointed out,

is that ADHD youngsters lack goal-directed persistence.[11] As Dr. Barkley explains it, those with ADHD have problems executing actions that involve forethought, planning, goal direction, self-discipline, willpower, and dogged persistence. Such people need to be taught the how-to's of self-regulation—especially by giving positive feedback and immediate rewards.

Adults with ADHD fail at work for the same reasons they struggled through school. They tend to lose jobs because they can't meet deadlines or prioritize tasks. You may have noticed that you have a hard time keeping your mind on one thing—unless it's something that absolutely fascinates you. When your boss is speaking to you, for example, you're already wondering if you'll have time to finish your work by five and what you should fix for dinner that night. For you, finishing anything is a chore because you get bored with a task after only a few minutes. Organization is difficult, too. So dinner probably won't turn out to be when or what you expected.

Frank Lee was well into his forties and his umpteenth sales job before he was diagnosed with ADHD. "I could not, for the life of me, finish a piece of paperwork," he says. "I was great at selling but terrible on follow-through."

The bright side of ADHD is that a lot of children, teens, and adults who have it not only learn to harness the energy and creativity that accompany it but often excel at certain endeavors, like sales. In fact, during a speech in 1994, Patricia H. Latham, J.D., explained that while an ADHD person has deficits, the disorder can also result in some traits—such as high energy, intensity, an affinity for stimulation, creativity, and colorfulness—that can be assets in the right job. "Certain types of work seem to work better for ADD adults," Latham said. "Sales, lobbying and promoting involve energy, innovation and social interaction. They offer stimulation and immediate feedback and rewards. A salesman makes a sale, it feels good. He gets something right away."[12]

HYPERACTIVITY

A hyperactive person is easy to spot. "Brian Donnelly," for example, was the most animated kid in his second-grade class. If he wasn't walking around talking to his classmates, he was staring out the window or watching the fish tank—always in motion. His energy was boundless, but rarely constructive.

For hyperactive children, the classroom is torment. They squirm in their seats, wiggle their feet, touch, tap, and fidget. In severe cases they are so incessantly energetic, they seem literally to bounce off the walls. As the mother of nine-year-old Anna Alden recalls, in kindergarten, "Anna would jump out of her seat and out the door. She used the hallways like a racetrack."

Teenagers and adults who are hyperactive often describe themselves as feeling incredibly restless both day and night. "There were days when I know I never sat down," says Susan Phillips. "But at bedtime, instead of being tired, I just couldn't turn it off. I couldn't sleep."

Several studies have found that children with ADHD have a higher likelihood of sleep problems than non-ADHD children.[13] There are two prominent theories as to why. One is that ADHD sufferers may also experience more sleep-related breathing disorders, such as snoring, mouth breathing, and pauses during sleep.[14] The second is that ADHD can be viewed as a chronic state of hyperarousal that results in those afflicted having greater difficulty settling down to sleep and staying in a deep sleep pattern.[15]

IMPULSIVITY

Children and adolescents with ADHD often fail to consider the potentially negative, destructive, or even life-threatening consequences that may result from some of their actions. They seem to engage in frequent, unnecessary risk-taking. Many tend to have an impossible time grasping the concept of thinking before acting.[16] Their inability to weigh the consequences of their actions can be detrimental, even deadly.

In the very young child, hitting, biting, and pinching are typical displays of impulsive behavior. Running into the street without looking is not so typical—and obviously more dangerous. And consider the kind of risks that Brian Donnelly, now 15, would take: "I was at this party," he recalls, "and got the bright idea of pouring lighter fluid on my gym shoes and then I lit them on fire. I was dancing around in the dark, and it was cool."

He recognizes that setting his shoes on fire could have hurt him. "But sometimes," Brian says, "I just do things."

ADHD Subtypes

Most people with ADHD have symptoms of inattentiveness, hyperactivity, and impulsivity, but sometimes the pattern isn't obvious. In the current edition of the American Psychiatric Association's *Diagnostic and Statistical Manual of Mental Disorders*, three subtypes of ADHD are offered: ADHD, Combined; ADHD, Predominantly Inattentive; and ADHD, Predominantly Hyperactive–Impulsive.

In order to diagnose any of the three subtypes, the symptoms have to be present for at least six months, and at least some of the inattentive, hyperactive, or impulsive symptoms that cause impairment must have been present prior to age seven.[17]

By the time ADHD patients reach adulthood, most have disciplined themselves enough to control physically destructive or dangerous impulses. Risk-taking behavior, though, often persists, usually in the guise of a personal or professional gamble that can interfere with a marriage or a career.

DIAGNOSTIC CRITERIA FOR ADHD SUBTYPES*

ADHD/Predominantly Hyperactive-Impulsive

A. Six or more of the following symptoms of **Hyperactivity-Impulsivity** have been present for at least six months to a degree that is maladaptive and inconsistent with developmental level:

1. Hyperactivity:

a. Often fidgets with hands or feet or squirms in seat.

b. Often leaves seat in classroom or in other situations in which remaining seated is expected.

c. Often runs about or climbs excessively in situations in which it is inappropriate (in adolescents or adults, may be limited to subjective feelings of restlessness).

d. Often has difficulty playing or engaging in leisure activities quietly.

e. Is often "on the go" or often acts as if "driven by a motor."

f. Often talks excessively.

2. Impulsivity:

a. Often blurts out answers before questions have been completed.

b. Often has difficulty awaiting turn.

c. Often interrupts or intrudes on others (e.g., butts into conversations or games).

*Reprinted with permission from the Diagnostic and Statistical Manual of Mental Disorders, Fourth Edition. Copyright 1994 American Psychiatric Association.

DIAGNOSTIC CRITERIA FOR ADHD SUBTYPES

ADHD/Predominantly Hyperactive-Impulsive *(continued)*

B. Some hyperactive-impulsive symptoms that caused impairment were present before age seven years.

C. Some impairment from the symptoms is present in two or more settings (e.g., at school and work; or at home and school).

D. There must be clear evidence of clinically significant impairment in social, academic, or occupational functioning.

ADHD/Predominantly Inattentive

A. Six or more of the following symptoms of **Inattention** have been present for at least six months and to a degree that is maladaptive and is inconsistent with the developmental level:

   1. Often fails to give close attention to details or makes careless mistakes in schoolwork, work, or other activities.

   2. Often has difficulty sustaining attention in tasks or play activities.

   3. Often does not seem to listen when spoken to directly.

   4. Often does not follow through on instructions and fails to finish schoolwork, chores, or duties in the workplace (not due to oppositional behavior or failure to understand instructions).

   5. Often has difficulties organizing tasks and activities.

6. Often avoids, dislikes, or is reluctant to engage in tasks that require sustained mental effort (such as schoolwork or homework).

7. Often loses things necessary for tasks or activities (e.g., toys, school assignments, pencils, books, or tools).

8. Is often distracted by extraneous stimuli.

9. Is often forgetful in daily activities.

B. Some inattentive symptoms that caused impairment were present before age seven years.

C. Some impairment from the symptoms is present in two or more settings (e.g., at school and work; or at home and school).

D. There must be clear evidence of clinically significant impairment in social, academic, or occupational functioning.

ADHD/Combined Type

A. Six or more of the following symptoms of **Inattention** have been present for at least six months and to a degree that is maladaptive and is inconsistent with the developmental level:

1. Often fails to give close attention to details or makes careless mistakes in schoolwork, work, or other activities.

2. Often has difficulty sustaining attention in tasks or play activities.

3. Often does not seem to listen when spoken to directly.

DIAGNOSTIC CRITERIA FOR ADHD SUBTYPES

ADHD/Combined Type *(continued)*

4. Often does not follow through on instructions and fails to finish schoolwork, chores, or duties in the workplace (not due to oppositional behavior or failure to understand instructions).

5. Often has difficulties organizing tasks and activities.

6. Often avoids, dislikes, or is reluctant to engage in tasks that require sustained mental effort (such as schoolwork or homework).

7. Often loses things necessary for tasks or activities (e.g., toys, school assignments, pencils, books, or tools).

8. Is often distracted by extraneous stimuli.

9. Is often forgetful in daily activities.

B. Six or more of the following symptoms of **Hyperactivity-Impulsivity** have been present for at least six months to a degree that is maladaptive and inconsistent with developmental level:

1. Hyperactivity:

a. Often fidgets with hands or feet or squirms in seat.

b. Often leaves seat in classroom or in other situations in which remaining seated is expected.

c. Often runs about or climbs excessively in situations in which it is inappropriate (in adolescents or adults, may be limited to subjective feelings of restlessness).

d. Often has difficulty playing or engaging in leisure activities quietly.

e. Is often "on the go" or often acts as if "driven by a motor."

f. Often talks excessively.

2. Impulsivity:

a. Often blurts out answers before questions have been completed.

b. Often has difficulty awaiting turn.

c. Often interrupts or intrudes on others (e.g., butts into conversations or games).

B. Some hyperactive-impulsive symptoms that caused impairment were present before age seven years.

C. Some impairment from the symptoms is present in two or more settings (e.g., at school and work; or at home and school).

D. There must be clear evidence of clinically significant impairment in social, academic, or occupational functioning.

Social Effects of ADHD

More than half of the children and an untold number of adults with ADHD have social difficulties. These are usually evidenced in peer relationships that are strained or, in some cases, nonexistent. They are observed both at work and at play.[18]

Young children with ADHD have trouble staying with one activity for an extended time and shift their attention not only from one toy or game to the next, but from one playmate to the next. As a result, they often have few opportunities to make meaningful attachments.

ADHD children talk more but are less efficient in organizing and communicating information to their friends. They are good conversationalists but poor listeners. And they can alienate others with behavior that seems inappropriate. Eric Spencer, for example, couldn't resist touching or poking other kids. As a result, his classmates often didn't like him.

In general, ADHD children are more aggressive, disruptive, domineering, intrusive, and noisy than other children. This is especially true for the boys, who tend to have more pronounced ADHD behaviors. Aggressive children often interpret the actions of others as hostile and respond accordingly. Fighting is the unfortunate result.

Aggressiveness colors their interactions with adults as well. ADHD children often display greater degrees of oppositional and defiant behavior and conduct problems, especially within the family. These problems compound the effects of ADHD and require specialized treatment programs. (These issues are dealt with in Chapters 10 and 11.)

Adults with ADHD can experience all of the same complications, which may jeopardize their marriages, friendships, and even jobs. The social problems of ADHD sufferers, persistently battering the psyche, often translate into psychological problems such as long-term lack of self-esteem. Depression and anxiety are typical results.

By the time he was in junior high school, Tim Gabriel was severely depressed. "In grade school I had no friends, only enemies," he says. His classmates, he remembers, would taunt him because they thought he was stupid. The worst part, he says, "is that when they called me a wimp, or a creep, or told me I was gross, I believed them."

Frank Lee spent his whole life listening to others tell him that he had "more potential." But "I was always thinking I was just plain stupid," he says. He failed both to excel as a student and to prosper in a career. Only in middle age was he diagnosed with ADHD.

Tim and Frank are both reaching their potentials now, but they are also being treated for depression.

Assessing and addressing ADHD early and effectively can help minimize or prevent social, academic, professional, and psychological consequences. That's what we'll discuss in Chapter 4, but first let's examine what is known about the causes of ADHD.

CHAPTER THREE

Was It Something I Did? The Causes of ADHD

"Your child *has* a problem."

"Your child *is* a problem."

What parent can bear to hear these words? Even if you know, deep down, that something just isn't right, when you get the verdict from a teacher or a pediatrician, your hunch becomes a reality that you have to face.

Finally.

It can almost be a relief to know that your child has a definite disorder with a name and with the hope of treatment.

But still, being human, you can't resist thinking, "What did I do wrong?"

The answer is nothing. You didn't cause your child or adolescent to have ADHD. You are no more responsible for it than you are for his asthma, diabetes, or allergies.

Although the symptoms of ADHD are behavioral and not physical, the disorder—like asthma, diabetes, and allergies—does have a distinct physiological origin. And like each of them, your child's likelihood of developing it is genetically determined, entirely beyond your control. It is a myth that poor parenting causes ADHD—just one of many myths about the disorder that has been propagated through the years and that has failed to be borne out by scientific research.[1]

The Making of Myths

The myths about ADHD really began in the early 1970s when a quiet, unassuming physician by the name of Benjamin Feingold became a virtual guru for frustrated parents of children with ADHD. For thousands of them, his claim that diet had a direct affect on behavior—particularly hyperactivity in children—was a godsend. The elixir he offered—dietary change—was completely natural, painless, and relatively inexpensive.[2]

Feingold's book, *Why Your Child Is Hyperactive*, and the controversies it stirred up led to considerable research into the causes of ADHD. Some theorists came along suggesting that refined sugar could cause ADHD.[3] But when C. Keith Conners, professor of medical psychology at Duke University Medical Center, studied the effects of diet, especially sugar, on behavior, his findings indicated that the effects of sugar vary with most children—whether or not they have ADHD—depending upon the carbohydrates and protein present in a previous meal that the child consumed.[4]

Still, parents have wanted to believe in the claims of Feingold and others because their theories provided easy, definitive answers. A groundswell of support escalated into a movement and eventually into the international Feingold Society. This organization, known in this country as the Feingold Associations of the United States, encourages the restriction of artificial flavorings, preservatives, and sugars in the diet.[5] Cutting back on the chemicals and empty calories we consume makes good sense, for just about anyone. That alone is enough to explain why the Feingold Society still exists today. But since the Feingold fervor of the 1970s, the fact that diet simply isn't a cause of ADHD has been proven time and time again, which explains why the degree of enthusiasm for the cause has been drastically diminished.[6]

Indeed, considerable research has refuted Feingold's theories. A 1983 report in the *Journal of the American Dietetic Association* said the diet was futile against ADHD. Morris A. Lipton, M.D. and James P. Mayo, M.D., wrote that the success rate of the diet was 1.5 percent at most. "The behavioral changes we note have nothing to do with the additives," Lipton said. "If there was any improvement at all, it may be attributed to the shift of the family focus on the child who causes changes in the way the entire family ate. It's purely psychological."[7]

Another study published in 1984 by Judith Rapoport, the chief of the Child Psychiatry Division of the National Institute of Mental Health, and her associates, examined boys who were said to be "sugar reactive" by their parents. Some of the twenty-one children in this group were given a sugar solution, while others received a placebo. On three different occasions, they were given physical, psychological, and behavioral evaluations.

The only significant treatment effect the researchers found was a slight *decrease* of motor activity among both ADHD and non-ADHD children.[8] One possible reason for this unexpected finding was that the study did not consider the age of the children. What this may mean is that diet and behavior are much more complex issues than is generally thought.

A similar study was carried out at the famed Menninger Clinic in Topeka, Kansas, and reported in the 1994 *Journal of Abnormal Psychology*. This study involved thirty-one sets of mothers and sons. The mothers believed that their children, all between the ages of five and seven, were adversely affected by eating sugar. The boys were divided randomly into two groups. In one group the mothers were told that their sons had been given a flavored drink with large amounts of sugar. In the other group the mothers were told their sons were given drinks with NutraSweet and that the artificial sweetener had no ill affect on a child's behavior.[9]

Despite the fact all the children drank the same artificially sweetened drink, only the mothers who believed their sons had ingested sugar reported a notable increase in the boys' activity levels.

These are just two of the many studies that have been performed in an attempt to identify a connection between diet and hyperactive or inattentive behaviors.[10] The results are consistent: No significant effect from food or beverages can be detected for ADHD children.[11]

Recently researchers have theorized that either asthma or some of the medications associated with it (such as theophylline) cause ADHD. A 1996 article in the *Journal of Attention Disorders* reviewed all the research and literature relating to asthma and asthma treatment. The authors concluded that asthmatic children are no more likely to have ADHD than are non-asthmatic children.[12]

Although some asthma medications may increase a child's activity level and decrease his or her attention span, these symptoms abate as soon as the medication is discontinued. Such temporary behavioral changes are rarely associated with long-term problems such as ADHD.[13]

Other suspected culprits in ADHD include prolonged labor, cesarean delivery, and the use of the drug pitocin during labor to stimulate contractions. Some doctors and parents have even hypothesized that yeast infections, inner-ear infections, and vitamin deficiencies cause ADHD.[14]

Brain infections, trauma during pregnancy, and

complications or injury during delivery have also been proposed as possible causes of ADHD. Some studies do show that certain types of brain damage are associated with ADHD.[15] But most ADHD children and adults do not have a history of brain injury or other brain trauma, either before or after birth.[16]

The Genetic Link

The most convincing research so far on the causes of ADHD points to a genetic, not an environmental basis. This research indicates that ADHD may be linked with a gene that regulates the action of norepinephrine and dopamine, chemicals manufactured in the brain.[17] "We haven't bagged the gene," says Dr. Edwin Cook, a child psychiatrist and molecular biologist who has led a research team at the University of Chicago. "But we've found a marker—a stretch of DNA—that when inherited with the gene confers susceptibility to ADHD."[18]

Frank Lee says it's obvious to him now that ADHD is a Lee family trait. "The Lee men have freckles, and the Lee men have ADHD," he says. But none of the Lee men knew they had ADHD until Frank's son, "Matt," was diagnosed. And even then it took a while to sink in: "We were so worried about Matt and what kind of treatment to try, we didn't see the big picture."

Within a year of Matt's diagnosis, Frank was also diagnosed. He learned enough about the disorder to be reasonably certain it had also affected his father and his grandfather. "I wish we could have known before," he says. "I feel bad that it took three generations to figure it out. I feel bad that Matt wound up with something that I probably passed along to him. But mostly I'm glad that finally we have ways to deal with it."

The genetic explanation was initially suggested by statistics that indicate that adults and children with ADHD have more relatives with the disorder than non-ADHD adults and children. If you have ADHD yourself, there's at least a 33 percent chance that one of your children also will be diagnosed.[19] If you and your spouse both have ADHD, the chance increases.[20] If you are a twin, the chances range from 75 to 91 percent that if one of you has ADHD, the other will, too.[21]

The New Technology

New tools and techniques for studying the brain may offer even more stunning discoveries about ADHD's origins. Already sophisticated X-ray studies like CAT (computerized axial tomography) and MRI (magnetic resonance imaging) scans show that the brains of people with ADHD do have distinctive differences from those of others. In the future we may be able to design treatments that can "repair" more specific areas and functions of the brain. With new complex scanners (like positron emission tomography, or PET scanning), we can actually measure the metabolic functioning of the brain, along with its structure, and so perhaps we'll come to see not only where the ADHD brain differs but how differently it works.

Advances in genetic mapping are bringing us closer than ever to discovering the exact genetic defect that causes ADHD.[22] A simple blood test to determine whether a child has the specific ADHD gene may well be developed, along with treatments that could genetically reengineer the defective DNA.

Clearly, new technology holds tremendous promise for ADHD treatments, but there is still much to learn. Compared with what experts know about the human heart, for example, our understanding of the brain is still rudimentary. Not only are the brain's functions extremely complex, but they vary greatly among individuals. For example, one person watching a particular movie may be moved to tears, while another may find humor in the same story. As we continue to study the brain, our new discoveries, not surprisingly, will lead to new questions.

Where, in the vastness of this phenomenon called the brain, does ADHD begin, what are the mechanisms that cause it, and how can it be repaired? To understand the enormity of the challenge these questions pose for researchers, let's look at what we do know about the brain.

What Is the Brain?

The brain is about the size of two fists and weighs about as much as a head of cabbage, yet it can store millions of bits of information. It's made up of many intricately entwined, fragile structures, each with a specific function. Together they accomplish processes of unfathomable complexity and power. Even the most sophisticated computer simply regurgitates information; only the human brain can initiate a new thought or experience an emotion. The brain is also amazing in its ability to grow and adapt to new situations.

The anatomy of the brain reflects our evolution. As our species transformed and our needs changed—to speak, to walk erect, to cultivate crops—the brain had to adapt itself. It met these challenges by manufacturing new structures—each one more complex—over the existing framework, literally developing from the inside out. It is now a highly organized structure made up of three distinct sections—the brain stem, the cerebellum, and the cerebral cortex—each having unique, specialized functions.

The *brain stem*, the most primitive section, is positioned deep within the skull. Very similar in appearance and function to a reptile's brain, it controls our basic biological functions, such as breathing, heart rate, body temperature, and blood pressure. Without any conscious effort, the brain stem tirelessly performs these functions, and it's a good thing it does—how could we ever sleep if we had to constantly remember to breathe?

The *cerebellum*, a considerable step up the evolutionary ladder, is a small gray structure that covers the brain stem like a mushroom cap. This portion of the brain coordinates more complex, purposeful movements like drinking a glass of water or hitting a golf ball.

The *cerebral cortex*, located on the outer portion of the brain, developed most recently. This structure is by far the most complex. While the other parts of the brain are more task-oriented, the cerebral cortex is designed to deal with behaviors and concepts. This high-functioning machine regulates our emotions and determines our personality. This portion of the brain is divided into two halves, or hemispheres. The hemispheres communicate with each other through a thick band of nerves called the corpus callosum. Each hemisphere is subdivided into four lobes—the occipital, the parietal, the temporal, and the frontal (or forebrain)—and each lobe has a different job.

The *occipital lobes* are located at the rear of the brain and have the job of processing all visual information. The eyes send optical images to this region to be analyzed. The result is that we are able to see. Injuries to the occipital lobe can impair vision or even cause blindness.

The *parietal lobes* are located in the center of each hemisphere of the cortex. They sense touch from every part of the body and control voluntary muscle movements. This area is often affected when a person experiences a stroke, resulting in a loss of feeling or ability to move parts of their bodies.

The *temporal lobes* are located just above the brain stem and are responsible for processing sounds and generating speech. Other areas in the temporal lobes function as memory storage. There is evidence that poor short-term memory, a major problem for children and adults with ADHD, may be due to dysfunction in the temporal lobes.

The *frontal lobes (forebrain)*, located just behind the forehead, are assigned the job of filtering stimulation. The brain is constantly being bombarded with so much data that it could easily become overwhelmed with electrical signals. Consider what happens, for instance, when you do something as simple as stepping out of your front door. Your senses are instantly flooded with hundreds, perhaps thousands of stimuli—from the sight of the blue sky to the sound of a dog barking to the smell of flowers. Yet somehow you are able to concentrate on one little bird sitting on the fence.

You can thank the forebrain for this incredible aptitude. Miraculously, it has the ability to process all the stimuli, weed out those that are extraneous and assign priorities to those that aren't. The important signals are then sent along to the other parts of the brain to be acted upon.

Sometimes the forebrain doesn't do a very good job of filtering the information. Children and adults with ADHD are extremely distracted by irrelevant stimuli, which renders them unable to concentrate.

This doesn't mean that these people have "broken frontal lobes"—it simply means that the lobes do not have the ability to prioritize data, and thus the individual is unable to focus. No wonder researchers suspect that forebrain malfunction may cause ADHD.

Consider some of the forebrain's other jobs. It is critical, for example, in organizing, completing, and comprehending complex actions. When you clean the garage, you must first take the car out, then sweep, move things around, and then replace the car. Those with ADHD are unable to complete such multistep tasks. They may take the car out and start to sweep. But then they may find their old bike and start to clean it up or take it for a ride. The job of cleaning the garage gets forgotten. One of the hallmarks of ADHD is the inability to make a plan and stick to it.

"My husband would decide to wash the windows thirty minutes before our dinner reservations," says "Jean McIntyre," the leader of an attention deficit support group. "It sounds funny, but when it happens day after day, it becomes a serious problem."

Another crucial forebrain function is to appraise whether an event is life-threatening. This is known as the "fight or flight" reaction. When you are confronted with a dire circumstance, the brain must quickly decide how you should react: Should you stand still and face the consequences, or should you run away? The forebrain assesses all the variables related to the threat, sets priorities, and tells the rest of the brain how to handle the situation. Children and adolescents with ADHD, more often than adults, are unable to prioritize these perils and often engage in dangerous activities without considering the consequences. Playing with matches and riding a bike down a steep hill don't seem like dangerous activities to many children with ADHD. They have a tendency to leap before they look.

The forebrain is also involved in such complex skills as writing and speaking. It coordinates hand-to-eye movements with other lobes. It isn't uncommon for children with ADHD to suffer from handwriting or fine motor problems.

Other functions performed by the frontal lobes are constantly being discovered. Because of its front-and-center position as well as its multifaceted abilities, this portion of the brain can easily be compared to the conductor of an orchestra. It interprets the music and directs the other lobes on how and when to play. When the conductor falls down on the job, the whole performance suffers.

Corresponding with Our Brain

The forebrain may be *where* a person with ADHD is affected, but researchers must also ask *how*. The brain performs its myriad functions by means of *neurons*. There are more than one hundred billion of these cells in the brain. They have the unique capacity to communicate with each other by way of an electrical charge. The gaps between neurons, over which they have to "shout" to communicate, are called *synapses*.

To communicate, neurons release tiny amounts of chemicals called *neurotransmitters* that jump across the synapse from one neuron to the next. The electric signal is then continued in the second neuron. Thus, the synapses function as tiny traffic lights for the signals as they reach the end of the neuron. The synapse must quickly decide whether to send the signal to nerve A, nerve B, or nerve C, or to all of them, or to stop the signal altogether. And it must make that decision in less than a hundredth of a second.

Two important neurotransmitters, dopamine and norepinephrine, are found throughout the brain, but they appear in abnormal levels in the frontal lobes of individuals with ADHD.[23] The reason for this phenomenon is unclear, but it is a consistent finding and is genetically determined.

The Brain and ADHD

It is increasingly evident that forebrain and synaptic dysfunction are responsible for the symptoms of ADHD.

• Using PET scanning, researchers have discovered that individuals with ADHD use less glucose in the forebrain—the area that affects certain thinking tasks. Glucose is the brain's main source of energy. If a person uses less glucose, it suggests they have less brain activity.[24]

• People with ADHD also have less activity in the left frontal and left parietal areas of the brain—the areas that affect concentration abilities—compared to people without ADHD. These findings, reported in 1995 by the University of Kansas Medical Center, were made by using another sophisticated X-ray technique known as SPECT (single photo emission computer tomography).[25]

• The volume of parts of the brain is also different in people who have ADHD. This difference has been demonstrated in research using MRI techniques. In 1996 the Child Psychiatry Division of the NIMH reported on a study it did with MRI in the journal *Archives of General Psychiatry*. ADHD subjects in this study had significantly smaller areas of the brain than patients without the disorder.[26]

These findings are significant not only in the study of ADHD but in the study of Tourette's syndrome as well, and they may suggest why there is a significant relationship between them.

TOURETTE'S SYNDROME

Tourette's syndrome is characterized by *tics*—repetitive behaviors such as blinking or twitching. Most of us have tics at one time or another, and most are benign and go away quickly. In the case of Tourette's syndrome—a complex and rare disorder—they persist and are often quite pronounced.

One study, reported in the *Journal of the American Academy of Child Psychiatry* in 1984, indicated that 62 percent of males under the age of 21 who were initially diagnosed with Tourette's could also be diagnosed with ADHD.[27] Other studies have confirmed that youngsters with ADHD often develop the kinds of tics seen in Tourette's syndrome.[28]

Evidence from genetic studies suggests that Tourette's syndrome is inherited. Having the gene that causes Tourette's may not result in a full-blown case of tics, but it does predispose an individual to the disorder. A person with the predisposition may have mild tics, an obsessive-compulsive disorder, or ADHD with few tics. It's also quite possible that the gene-carrying person may not develop Tourette's at all.[29]

The leading research on Tourette's is being carried out at the National Institute of Neurological Disorders and Stroke, a part of the National Institutes of Health in Bethesda, Maryland. Current studies are exploring how neurotransmitters may be involved in Tourette's syndrome.[30] Some of the research findings indicate that for both ADHD and Tourette's, there are abnormal dopamine levels, increased right frontal brain activities, and decreased volume of the brain.[31] This commonality strongly suggests that as advances are made in the search for causes and improved treatment of both ADHD and Tourette's, findings in one area may well apply to the other.

There has been concern in the past that treatment of ADHD with Ritalin *caused* Tourette's syndrome in some children and adolescents. But, more and more experts, after reviewing the latest research studies, have concluded that, in the reported cases, Ritalin was almost certainly triggering symptoms that had been dormant and would have appeared sooner or later. The most recent research suggests that proper dosages of Ritalin and other medications for ADHD may even result in decreased tics in patients with Tourette's.[32]

This indicates that if you have or your child has both ADHD symptoms and tics, you can consider Ritalin a relatively safe and effective medication.

The Brain and Ritalin

Stimulant medications such as Ritalin affect the brain of a person with ADHD differently from the way they would affect the brain of a person without the disorder. Specifically, they alter the levels of the neurotransmitters dopamine and norepinephrine, chemicals that tend to be low in individuals with ADHD. It is by correcting the levels of dopamine and norepinephrine that Ritalin, in proper doses, can often improve ADHD symptoms.[33]

As a parent of an ADHD child, your feelings of guilt are natural. But they are clearly not warranted: Much research and investigation have proven that ADHD is physiological.

ADHD's presence is beyond your control. But the treatment is within your grasp.

CHAPTER FOUR

The ADHD Assessment

*U*ntil the day when ADHD can be diagnosed by a simple blood test—or when PET scans, CAT scans, and MRIs are more practical and easier to interpret—the best means we have to determine whether someone has the disorder is a multilevel assessment: a series of behavioral and medical evaluations. Unlike a medical diagnosis, which offers a conclusion based on concrete data—an X ray, for instance—an assessment offers a judgment based on subjective data, such as a personality profile. While it's certainly not as cut-and-dried as a medical diagnosis, an assessment certainly isn't invasive or painful, and in most cases it doesn't have to be costly.

It does have to be time-consuming, though, and if it's not, you should be suspicious about its accuracy.

"What concerns me," says Robert Resnick, Ph.D.,[1] "is when a fifteen-minute interview in a doctor's office leads to an attention deficit diagnosis." Resnick, director of the Attention Deficit Disorder Clinic at the Medical College of Virginia Commonwealth University and past president of the American Psychological Association, estimates that the average pediatrician spends "twelve minutes" with a youngster in making an ADHD assessment.

The Importance of the Assessment

The ideal ADHD assessment includes an initial screening and comprehensive evaluations by at least three experts—physicians, psychologists, social workers, or educators—who are authorities on ADHD. An initial screening serves as a filtering process to determine whether evidence of ADHD is sufficient to suggest further assessment. This screening will determine whether the behaviors the person is displaying are characteristic of ADHD and whether they are being displayed at a developmentally inappropriate level or to a problematic degree. Psychological clinics are the typical settings for these initial interviews, although many pediatricians and family physicians are qualified to administer them. Obviously the patient is the primary focus of the screening, but parents and spouses are also an integral part of the process.

Why is a thoroughgoing assessment so important?

Consider the experience of "Gina Lovett." When her three-year-old son began waking the entire family in the middle of the night with loud tantrums and destructive behavior, Gina turned to her pediatrician—a kind, gentle man who had treated her family for two generations. "Two minutes after that doctor walked in the room, he handed me a prescription for Ritalin," she says.

Gina was disappointed *and* suspicious. Instead of filling the prescription, she began searching for a new doctor. "I was familiar with Ritalin," Gina says, "and I wasn't comfortable about giving it to a toddler— especially when the doctor hadn't even made eye contact with him."

In record time Gina's doctor had made a multitude of mistakes. For starters, Ritalin is rarely recommended for children younger than five. It's also inadvisable to prescribe any psychostimulant without performing at least a rudimentary psychological evaluation. But perhaps the most surprising error Gina's doctor made—he is now, incidentally, her ex-doctor—was assuming on the basis of a single symptom that the boy had ADHD. "He never asked me one question," Gina says. "Just grunted and started scribbling."

Gina's toddler eventually outgrew his nocturnal outbursts, and she now attributes them to night terrors—a phenomenon she learned about from her new pediatrician. Had she not followed her instincts, her son would have been exposed to all the risks of the drug without realizing the benefits.

A proper screening may disclose other, serious disorders that mimic ADHD but require radically different treatments.

"Mitchell Olsen" took Ritalin for three years until
his third-grade teacher finally pressed the issue and
convinced Mitchell's mother, "Anita," that she should
have him assessed. "I didn't even know there was such
a thing as an assessment," says Anita. "I just trusted
the doctor who gave us the medication."

Mitchell, it turns out, is dyslexic—he does not
have ADHD. He is now getting help for his severe
reading disability, and is doing well at school. But,
those three years took their toll. "He went through so
much failure and embarrassment," Anita says, "he's
got a real inferiority complex."

After battling agitation and sleep problems for
much of her life, "Connie Wilson," 28, finally went to
see a doctor about it. "I lost weight and had headaches," she says, "and I slept even worse." The doctor
thought her symptoms were related to ADHD and
prescribed Ritalin.

A second doctor whom Connie consulted recommended an assessment. This assessment led to a diagnosis of depression. Wellbutrin, an antidepressant, and
psychotherapy have worked wonders for her.

Unfortunately, hasty diagnoses of ADHD are not
just perpetuated by a few bad apples in the medical
profession but are extremely common. Teachers and
school counselors—who are critical to the proper assessment and treatment of ADHD children and often
initiate the process—sometimes use skimpy, checklist-

style screening tools to identify affected students. The parents and physicians typically see only the results, not the inadequate testing method.

"Lisa Peters" was a little too rambunctious as far as her first-grade teacher was concerned. The six-year-old chattered incessantly and couldn't seem to concentrate on her assignments. "The teacher sent home a one-paragraph letter to give to our doctor saying that Lisa probably had ADHD," says Lisa's father, "John." "It worried us, and so we began the process."

They started with the psychologist in their school district—and that is also where they stopped. Lisa, it turned out, was intelligent and bored, and to top things off, she needed glasses. An accelerated grade-school class and a visit to an optometrist made a world of difference.

Even the media have jumped on the ADHD band-wagon. During an eleven P.M. newscast in Detroit, a two-minute test was given to help viewers determine "if you suffer from ADHD"—as if any disorder could be diagnosed from a TV quiz. ADHD has become such a well-known syndrome that people almost seem to have lost sight of the fact that it is a serious condition, needing proper diagnosis and treatment.

Looking for Help

How can the average person find professionals quali-fied to perform an ADHD assessment? If you don't have the luxury of a referral from a trusted friend or

family member, plenty of other resources can assist you
in finding the right person for the job.

ADHD SUPPORT GROUPS

CHADD (Children and Adults with Attention Deficit
Disorder) is the best known of these organizations.
Founded in 1987 by a group of parents and professionals, CHADD now has more than 32,000 members
in local chapters across the country. Meetings, held
monthly, are open to the general public, are free of
charge, and feature a wide range of expert speakers and
discussion topics. An extensive selection of literature
and handouts related to ADHD is almost always available. In addition, most CHADD groups will be able to
recommend professionals in your area whom the organization recognizes and supports.

To locate the CHADD chapter closest to you,
check for the listing in the business pages of your local
telephone directory. Or see the Resources section of
this book.

A SCHOOL COUNSELOR, TEACHER, OR PRINCIPAL

Most educational professionals have made it their business to learn as much as possible about ADHD. Start
by contacting your school district's board of education
office and ask them to point you in the right direction.
Many school districts employ psychologists, social
workers, and nurses. If yours does not, usually at least

one teacher in the district has specific ADHD experience and training. Chances are you won't be the first person seeking advice.

A QUALIFIED PEDIATRICIAN

Of course you could spend a lot of time checking credentials, but word of mouth is probably the best way to find a pediatrician. First, you should ask *your* doctor if he knows someone in the area. He may be able to suggest someone in the area whom he respects. If you attend a CHADD meeting, ask other parents for referrals.

A COMMUNITY MENTAL HEALTH AGENCY

Even if your local agency has no ADHD-trained psychologist or social worker on its staff, the odds are that someone there will be able to make a recommendation.

If you aren't satisfied with the results from any of these options, there are numerous other resources. They include:

• Private schools specializing in ADHD or learning disabilities

• College or university education or psychology departments

• University-affiliated hospitals

• Private psychological outpatient clinics (check your yellow pages, or call your local physician referral service)

• Educational therapists or learning specialists in private practice (ask at your child's school, check the yellow pages, or ask your pediatrician for a referral)

HOW DO YOU KNOW THE PROFESSIONAL IS QUALIFIED?

Plenty of doctors and psychologists consider themselves qualified to assess and treat ADHD simply on the basis of their general training, but you should look for professionals who have specialized training in ADHD.

Before you sign on, find out:

• If the professional has been involved in the assessment and treatment of ADHD in the past, and if so, for how long

• If the professional has had specialized training in the assessment and treatment of ADHD. Most physicians and psychologists will provide this information upon request. Ask a member of the office staff if a résumé or list of the professional's credentials is available, in writing. Otherwise, ask him or her in person.

• How the screening or assessment will be administered

• What tests or procedures will be used in the assessment

• How the professional feels about working with other professionals in making the diagnosis

• How long the process will take

• How you will be kept informed

• Whether the professional will be able to make recommendations for continuing treatment

• The costs of the entire evaluation and possible treatment (this will vary greatly depending on your insurance coverage, the type of evaluation performed, and the facility performing the service)

• Details about insurance coverage and payment plans

If the professional is hesitant to answer these questions, it's probably wise to move on. Remember, you're probably going to forge long-term relationships with many of the professionals who work with you on this evaluation. Feeling comfortable and confident is absolutely necessary to a positive outcome for you and for your child.

The ADHD Assessment

SCREENING INTERVIEWS

If the initial screening yields evidence of ADHD, a more intensive screening will be the first step in the

ADHD assessment. This screening typically involves an interview of both parent and child with a pediatrician or school psychologist, who may use questionnaires and checklists to evaluate the symptoms more carefully. It's important to understand that even when an interview is conducted by a qualified professional, it is not a substitute for a complete assessment. Jumping the gun at this point can result in a misdiagnosis or a missed diagnosis.

Screening questions might include queries about:

• School or job performance

• Family history of ADHD

• Sleep problems

• A recent stress, like death or divorce, in the family

• Any prior ADHD evaluation

If ADHD is suspected after the screening, more in-depth assessment interviews will take place.

JoAnne Evans, president of CHADD, says her organization supports multifaceted evaluations by a team of physicians and psychologists.[2] Many ADHD clinics, such as Robert Resnick's, also include educators in the diagnostic process.

An ADHD assessment for a child should include:

• A parent interview

• An educational assessment

A complete ADHD assessment for an adult or a child should also include:

• A personal interview

• A medical evaluation

• A psychological evaluation

THE PARENT INTERVIEW

The next thing the members of your assessment team need to do is to get to know your family better. You, of course, are their best source.

You'll be asked about your child's family and medical histories and behavioral background. A wise professional will rely heavily on the input of the people who spend the most time with the child—the parents. Parents observe the child's day-to-day behavior patterns in a consistent setting.

Since school problems are often associated with ADHD, you'll probably be questioned in depth about your perceptions of your youngster's academic difficulties and your expectations for achievement and behavior at school.

The questions you are asked will be designed to disclose any history of learning disabilities or psychiatric problems in your family. This information is important because of the genetic component of ADHD and related disorders. If they run in your family, you and your children are at increased risk.

You may also be asked whether you, or your spouse, have ever been depressed. Depression and ADHD have much in common, including the fact that they're both genetic.[3] They also tend to occur together, but because they have very similar symptoms, the depression is often masked by the ADHD (see Chapter 5).

Clinicians will also want to know about your child's prenatal history. Questions about pregnancy, physical care, and even maternal alcohol use during pregnancy will probably be posed. The reason for these questions is that some disorders caused by prenatal problems, such as anoxia (a lack of oxygen to the developing baby's brain) or toxoplasmosis (an in utero infection of the baby's brain) can mimic ADHD.

You may be uncomfortable with this kind of probing. When you're asked certain background questions, it may seem as though you're being blamed for your child's difficulties. If you feel this way, the best thing to do is to clear the air. Make sure you have an opportunity to discuss your feelings—and your fears. Anger and resentment will only get in the way of the information-gathering process and ultimately the valid assessment. Your honest answers may hold the key to the proper diagnosis.

The clinician conducting the personal interview may eventually want to speak with you and your child together to observe and assess your interactions. In the beginning most ADHD children are on their best behavior, but after they become more comfortable, they begin to exhibit some of the behaviors—such as increased activity, fidgeting, distractibility, and poor compliance—that can be useful in the assessment procedure. While such observations may not directly determine if ADHD is present, they are valuable when deciding on a treatment program, particularly when parents need assistance in managing difficult behavior.[4]

The experts will want to know about the discipline tactics used in your home. They'll also need to be informed about significant parental disagreements on child-rearing issues. (Obviously these issues become more complicated in cases of blended families and joint custody.)

Rating scales for parents

As part of an objective and comprehensive evaluation, you should also expect to be asked to complete standardized rating scales and checklists. Some of the most common evaluations include the Child Behavior Checklist—Parent Form and the Conners' Parent Rating Scale—Revised. Sometimes the Home Situations Questionnaire—Revised is used to ascertain more about the impact of the attention deficit problems on the family.

Rating scales are valuable because they allow parents to rate their child's behavior, and they give the clinician the opportunity to compare your response with those of other parents both with ADHD and non-ADHD children.

CONNERS' PARENT RATING SCALE—REVISED (S)[*]
BY C. KEITH CONNERS, PH.D.

Instructions: Below are a number of common problems that children have. Please rate each item according to your child's behavior in the last month. For each item, ask yourself, "How much a problem has this been in the last month?" and circle the best answer for each one. If none, not at all, seldom, or very infrequently, you would circle 0. If very much true, or it occurs very often or frequently, you would circle 3. You would circle 1 or 2 for ratings in between. Please respond to each item.

	NOT TRUE AT ALL	JUST A LITTLE TRUE	PRETTY MUCH TRUE	VERY MUCH TRUE
• Inattentive, easily distracted	0	1	2	3
• Difficulty doing or completing homework	0	1	2	3
• Short attention span	0	1	2	3
• Fidgets with hands or feet or squirms in seat	0	1	2	3
• Hard to control in malls or while grocery shopping	0	1	2	3
• Messy or disorganized at home or school	0	1	2	3

THE EDUCATIONAL ASSESSMENT

Although children with ADHD will usually display some or all of their symptoms prior to going to school, it's most often when a child *first* enters school that the seriousness of the symptoms is noted, typically by a teacher.

Teachers are somewhat more objective than parents, since they work with many children of the same age and can more readily identify behaviors that fall outside the norm. Teachers also have contact with children in many kinds of settings—the classroom, the hallway, the cafeteria, and on the playground—and so can see which situations are especially challenging for a specific child.

Rating scales for teachers

Besides giving their behavioral observations in an interview, teachers also can fill out a rating scale such as the Child Behavior Checklist, Teacher Report Form or the Conners' Teacher Rating Scale, Revised. The information provided not only allows the professional to assess the child's behavior in the classroom but is also useful in establishing a baseline for a later evaluation of the success of the treatment approach. These scales should be readily available to your child's teacher, and you should feel free to ask a teacher to fill them out.

School history

A detailed school history will also be essential to obtain a clear diagnosis of ADHD. Report cards, assignments, and written teacher evaluations are excellent indicators of the degree of difficulty the child has experienced in such areas as completing schoolwork, concentrating on tasks, controlling impulses, and focusing attention.[5]

THE PSYCHOLOGICAL EVALUATION AND PERSONAL INTERVIEW

Of all the aspects of the ADHD assessment, the psychological evaluation is often the most dreaded.

"I wasn't about to take my kid to a shrink," says "Joe Gallardo," whose daughter, "Maria," was in the fourth grade when she was suspected of having ADHD. Joe says he felt that the mere suggestion was an assault on his—and his daughter's—mental stability.

It was the family pediatrician who finally convinced Joe to go—or at least to send Maria with her mother. One of the standard tests was administered by the psychologist—the Wechsler Intelligence Scale for Children III—and the results indicated that Maria was extraordinarily intelligent. It was a valuable tool for the Gallardos to take to her school, where she had been having academic problems.

Unfortunately, Maria's strength had been buried by the fallout of ADHD. Her mind was high functioning but her ability to focus on schoolwork, homework, or any chore at hand was severely impaired. Treatment of the ADHD literally turned her life around.

Although some ADHD assessments do turn up psychological disorders, as a rule the psychologist's role in the diagnosis of ADHD is to observe and interpret the behaviors exhibited by you or your child. Like the medical examination, the psychological evaluation can help rule out other intellectual, academic, and emotional factors that could be causing the ADHD symptoms. Or, as in Maria's case, the psychological evaluation could discover an untapped strength.

Personal interview

The psychological evaluation should include a structured interview of you and your child that systematically poses questions about those areas of a person's life that are most likely to be affected by the symptoms of ADHD: school, work, family, and peer relationships. Such an interview will take, in most instances, about forty-five minutes.

Your perception, or your child's perceptions of the problem can be very helpful in the ADHD assessment procedure. Along with the symptoms, the clinician will want to know what emotions—such as anger, frustration, or depression—you or your child experience.

A psychologist's or physician's interview with the child will be used to gain a general impression of the youngster's appearance, language capabilities, and social skills. The expert will also work to establish a rapport with the child, which will be helpful in the treatment phase, after the diagnosis has been made. Children typically describe their problems as being less serious or severe than parents and teachers do. But the way a child characterizes social problems with peers or describes attention difficulties can be useful.

A child can also offer insights about a traumatic event that may have yielded behavioral difficulties and that may have been overlooked by, or be unknown to, parents and teachers. For example, a child might feel intense sibling rivalry, feel rejected or picked on by peers, or experience emotional or physical abuse at home.

Twelve-year-old "Christopher Beck" was suspected of having ADHD because he was bored and unmotivated in class. In addition, he frequently misplaced his homework or didn't complete it at all. During the initial interview with Christopher, the psychologist asked him about his relationships at home.

He eventually began describing the feelings he had for his stepfather, a man Christopher said was critical, verbally abusive, and punitive. "I hate him so much, I could kill him," Christopher said angrily. When Christopher told about being slammed into the wall on more than one occasion by the man, the psychologist filed a protective service report for abuse and began to advocate a move for the boy to his biological father's house in another state. Later, after this move was effected, Christopher's schoolwork and motivation improved markedly. The psychologist's interview was critical in establishing that Christopher's problem was not ADHD.

When an evaluation is being conducted with an older child or adolescent, the interviewer will certainly be interested in determining whether substance abuse problems are contributing to the child's condition.

If you're an adult being assessed for ADHD, the clinical interview will explore any problems you are having with work-related tasks, organizational skills, short-term memory, and ability to complete projects. The interview will provide you with a chance to describe the history of your symptoms as they evolved over time and affected your schooling, employment, and relationships.

Psychological tests

The psychological examiner may also administer a battery of psychological tests. Psychological tests are also important because when ADHD children are examined by a psychologist, they often display acceptable levels of attention and behavioral control. In the psychological interview, which is highly structured and involves one-to-one interaction, ADHD youngsters often look and act most attentively.[7] The test battery is selected to measure the ability to attend to and concentrate on tasks that resemble those typically affected by attention deficits.

Psychological testing often takes three hours or longer, and the cost of an evaluation may be several hundred dollars. Parents should make sure that the test battery includes most of the following tests. If an examiner plans to skip one or more of them or uses some others not listed here, you should ask for an explanation.

The test battery might include:

• *Wechsler Intelligence Scale for Children—Third Edition (WISC III).* This standardized test measures the child's verbal and performance (nonverbal) intelligence. The verbal portion measures abilities such as vocabulary, short-term memory, and commonsense reasoning. As an individual test administered verbally by the psychological examiner, its advantage is that no reading is involved.

• *The Bender Visual Motor Gestalt Test.* This test is a copying exercise designed to measure maturation of visual-perceptual and visual-motor functioning.

• *Developmental Test of Visual-Motor Integration.* This perceptual-motor test for children between the ages of four and thirteen years measures visual perception and fine motor skills. Children are required to copy up to twenty-four geometric designs. While ADHD children are not necessarily impaired in their perceptual-motor functioning, such youngsters often impulsively make errors or have unique responses to frustration while performing a drawing test.[8]

• *The Sentence Completion Test.* This test requires the child to finish a sentence (for example, "The best thing about school is . . ."). Designed to elicit responses from the child's underlying mental state, personality, and mood, this test offers an overall picture of adjustment.

• *Kinetic Family Drawing, Draw-A-Person Test, House-Tree-Person Test and Goodenough-Harris Drawing Test.* These tests discern a child's personality characteristics or underlying emotional problems through drawings of themselves or others.

• *Children's Apperception Test (CAT) or Roberts Apperception Test.* These personality tests require children to make up stories and answer questions about a series of pictures. Very often the stories that ADHD children tell have themes related to impulsive behavior and failures in learning.[9]

• *Rorschach Psychodiagnostic Test.* This is one of the best known of the projective tests, in use for nearly a century. The patient is shown a series of ten inkblots, one at a time, and is asked to interpret them. The test reveals personality factors and mood and psychological problems.

The standard psychological test battery, which implements all or most of those described above, is useful in determining the presence of learning disabilities or emotional problems. An adult being evaluated for ADHD will receive the adult versions of some of these tests, for instance, the WAIS—III (Wechsler Adult Intelligence Scale—Third Edition) instead of the WISC—III.

This standard test battery alone cannot reliably rule ADHD in or out. Recently developed tests have great potential as reliable components in a team assessment because they're more objective and less contingent on personal opinions of interviewers. Usually referred to as Continuous Performance Tests (CPT), these widely studied measures of vigilance, attention span, and concentration require a youngster to observe letters and numbers that are rapidly projected on a computer screen. The child is required to respond by pressing a space bar or mouse button when a certain stimulus appears. The score taps both sustained attention and impulse control.

Other Continuous Performance Tests that are extremely useful in determining the presence of ADHD include the Gordon Diagnostic System, the Conners' Continuous Performance Test, the Vigil Continuous Performance Test, and the Test of Variables of Attention (TOVA).[10]

The trained psychologist will also observe the process a child goes through to answer test questions and solve test items. This kind of information can be very helpful in making a conclusion about ADHD. For example, "Megan Johnson," a 14-year-old girl who had been struggling in school for several years, was evaluated by a psychologist to determine the presence of ADHD. During the testing procedure the psychologist noted that Megan made jokes when she couldn't recall instructions. When filling out a written questionnaire, she responded to questions impulsively, rarely taking the time to think through her answers. Sometimes she made up answers in order to avoid dealing with more difficult questions. In her report the psychologist wrote, "Megan's impulsive style strongly suggests ADHD and further indicates one of the reasons why homework is usually a weakness for her." Her impulsive style during the testing showed how she generally handled test-taking at school and perhaps homework as well, often resulting in errors. The psychologist recommended that as one approach to treatment, Megan be taught to slow down and complete homework and take tests with more deliberation.

THE MEDICAL EVALUATION

This component of the ADHD assessment is critically important for children and adults alike. A thorough medical evaluation may assist in the diagnosis of ADHD, or it may identify another medical condition that could be producing the symptoms.

"Jenny Boyd," a six-year-old in the first grade, seemed to be having problems staying involved during class. She was also unable to pay attention consistently. During a parent-teacher conference, her teacher told her mother that she thought the child had ADHD. Jenny's pediatrician, during a subsequent examination, found that the girl was experiencing petit mal seizures. They were eventually controlled with medication, and her attention lapses stopped.

Besides epilepsy, other physical problems such as middle ear infections, visual impairment, and hypoglycemia can produce ADHD-like symptoms.

Depending on the child's or adult's medical history, the doctor may perform such neurological exams as an electroencephalogram (EEG) to rule out a seizure disorder. More invasive tests, such as a CAT scan or MRI, are generally limited to patients who have obvious neurological problems, such as paralysis or tremors. Although, as we mentioned before, these tests can offer physical clues about ADHD, this diagnostic use for them is still considered experimental and has not been sanctioned by the medical community.[6]

Making the ADHD Diagnosis

In order to arrive at an ADHD diagnosis, the assessment team should collectively agree that the following statements are true about you or your child:

• There *are* persistent problems with inattentiveness, hyperactivity, and impulsivity to a degree that impairs daily functioning.

• The developmental or family history indicates significant evidence of ADHD symptoms.

• Teacher and parent rating scales indicate ADHD.

• ADHD symptoms are observed in diverse situations.

• The physical and psychological examinations fail to identify any other plausible reasons for the ADHD symptoms.

Only after such careful diagnosis is made can a treatment plan be developed. The plan might include a recommendation for medication, family therapy, parent training, and social skills treatment. For example,

Megan Johnson's psychologist came up with the following recommended treatment plan:

> It is recommended that Megan be considered for medical management to assist her in better focusing her attention. In addition, she should be referred for tutoring so that she has supportive help in improving her achievement while learning to slow down her style in responding to tests. Because of low self-esteem, she could benefit from psychotherapy that would assist her in achieving a more positive view of herself and her academic abilities. Finally, she and her parents should be involved in family therapy, which would help them learn to better handle her negative attitudes and oppositional behavior and at the same time help both Megan and her parents to communicate better.

The various components of treatment are discussed in later chapters.

CHAPTER FIVE

If It's Not ADHD, What Else Could It Be?

*U*nless you thought you or your child had attention deficit hyperactivity disorder, you probably wouldn't have gone through an assessment in the first place. Chances are you're pretty prepared for a positive diagnosis. It might even throw you if the assessment team determines that ADHD isn't the problem after all, or is only part of the problem. Sometimes other disorders mimic or appear along with ADHD, complicating matters and confusing the diagnosis. Some of these problems, such as depression, are relatively common, while others, such as Tourette's syndrome, are rare.[1]

Most of the related disorders are believed to have organic origins similar to those of ADHD. This helps to explain why they are often mistaken for each other and why they have a tendency to appear together.

Effective treatment is available for each of these disorders, and if any of them are suggested during the assessment, you should discuss follow-up with your physician or another member of the assessment team. The treatment usually involves a combination of medications and psychotherapy. Remember, you've already overcome the biggest hurdle—recognizing the problem in the first place.

These are some of the other disorders that might be diagnosed during an ADHD assessment.

Depression

Depression is one of the most overlooked medical problems, particularly in young children.[2] There are a number of reasons for this oversight.

First of all, the stereotype of depression as chronic sadness is misleading. Adults tend to internalize symptoms, while children tend to act them out. A depressed adult, for instance, might sleep a lot, while a depressed child might get in fights or stop doing schoolwork.

Sometimes depressed children go to great extremes to hide their symptoms. Young children are typically not good at expressing their feelings. They often don't know how to articulate their moods, or they downplay what they interpret as negative or "bad" feelings.

Then, too, feelings of depression may wax and wane and therefore aren't always evident, even to the affected individual.

Depressed children, especially those who are younger, are often pigeonholed as "sullen" or "serious" by their parents and family members. These adjectives are far less threatening than "depressed."

Today, fortunately, depression is being recognized and treated with increasing frequency. Public awareness and better diagnostic tools are partially responsible. Ironically, so is ADHD. As many as 70 percent of children with ADHD can also be diagnosed as clinically depressed at some point in their young lives, and the incidence of ADHD adults with depression is even greater.[3] Both ADHD and depression are genetic, both are neurochemical disorders, and both usually begin occurring early in life.

One of the primary manifestations of depression is an inability to concentrate.[4] Since that's one of the primary symptoms of ADHD too, it's easy to see why one might conceal or be mistaken for the other. Some other warning signs of depression are:

• A sadness, better described as a feeling of hopelessness, that lasts longer than a few days. This feeling may come and go.

• A sleep disorder—either too much sleep or not enough. Sleep problems are significant in distinguishing depression from ADHD. The sleep problems of ADHD children often are related to their attempts to get extra attention at bedtime and to early rising, instead of the insomnia that's seen in depression.[5]

• Poor appetite. Generally children or adolescents with ADHD have a good appetite.

• Fatigue or lethargy

• Low self-esteem

• Low energy and decreased motivation

• Decreased interest in activities

Anxiety Disorder

The symptoms of anxiety, like those of depression, may not necessarily be obvious. The anxious child or adult may appear to be entirely in control. Beneath the surface, however, she may be in emotional agony. Too often children and adults with anxiety disorder are brushed off as "high-strung" or "nervous." Children and adults who are anxious may experience concentration problems— also a hallmark of ADHD and depression.[6]

The following symptoms, particularly in children, could be indicative of anxiety disorder:

• Excessive nervousness

• Constant complaining about illnesses

• Extreme self-consciousness

- Restlessness

- Excessive worrying

Tourette's Syndrome

This unusual disorder—characterized by varying degrees of compulsive vocalizations, motor twitches, or both—has many points of correspondence with ADHD. Both of them, for instance, appear around the age of six or seven and sometimes diminish in early adulthood. Both run in families. The symptoms of each are worsened by stress, excitement, or anxiety. It's not surprising that some research has indicated that ADHD and Tourette's are basically the same biochemical malfunction, taken to varying degrees and exhibited in different ways.[7] Some practitioners contend that every person with Tourette's syndrome is also afflicted with ADHD.[8]

Whatever the case may be, the two disorders are so tightly bound together that it's caused some major difficulties in treating them. Ritalin, for instance, was blamed for years for causing tic disorders in children. Eventually it was determined that the drug triggered tics only in children with a predisposition to Tourette's. Now even that conclusion is questionable. Conflicting reports, based on recent studies, indicate that Ritalin may, in some cases, actually decrease tics.[9]

Clearly, any child with ADHD and a family history of Tourette's syndrome, or a present tic disorder, should be monitored closely.

Symptoms of Tourette's syndrome include:

• Facial or vocal tics, including coughing, eye-twitches, and grunting

• In more severe cases, the symptoms can progress to the neck, the arms, and occasionally the trunk and legs. They often involve repetitive motions, vocalizations, and twitches that worsen during times of stress or excitement.

• The most severe cases can involve vocalizations of phrases or vulgar obscenities.

Oppositional Defiant Disorder

Oppositional defiant disorder (ODD) in a child can be agonizing for parents. Most evidence indicates that ODD behaviors, seen predominantly in boys, are not genetic or neurochemical but environmental in origin.[10] Although children without ADHD certainly do exhibit oppositional defiant behavior, ADHD increases the probability that they will develop it and hastens the process.[11]

Oppositional defiant disorder is not simply a matter of whining, refusing to obey, or throwing a temper tantrum. It involves a consistent pattern of hostility and disregard for authority.

Possibly one of the first diagnostic clues to ODD is the child's attitude toward a parent. When a mother simply asks her child to sit down and is rejoined with a belligerent "shut up" and a swat, that's a clue. Of course, one incident isn't enough to go on, but it should at the least be a warning sign.

Symptoms include:

• Angry moods

• Chronic defiance

• Argumentativeness

• Negativism

Conduct Disorder

This serious personality disorder is characterized by a blatant defiance of rules. Criminal behavior and total disregard for the feelings or rights of others are generally hallmarks of this problem. It is highly unlikely that ADHD alone contributes to conduct disorder, nor has it ever been proven to be entirely either genetic or physiologically induced. Most experts agree that conduct disorder is a result of several environmental factors, not the least of which is a hostile family environment.[12] Conduct disorder is seldom diagnosed in young children, but sometimes it is diagnosed in children under age ten. Most often its onset occurs in late childhood and early adolescence.[13]

Symptoms include:

• Repetitive acts of aggression and violence

• Frequent contacts with police or legal authorities

• School or home truancy

• Chronic disobedience and rule violations at home

• Substance abuse (frequently associated with conduct disorder)

Substance Abuse

On the surface ADHD and substance abuse appear to have little in common. But the two disorders are similar in several ways. Among their shared characteristics are a predominance in males, a tendency to appear in individuals who are risk takers, and their appearance in conjunction with low self-esteem, depression, and ODD.

Although some symptoms of drug abuse—like slurred speech, bloodshot eyes, and needle marks— are obvious, many are subtle and are often perilously similar to the behavioral patterns of ADHD. These can include:

- Poor academic performance

- Inability to concentrate

- Hyperactivity

- Sleep disorders

Learning Disabilities

A learning disability is a specific problem that can impair a child's capacity to absorb and process information. A learning disabled child is often of average or above-average intelligence but lacks the ability to learn in one or more particular areas.

Learning disabilities are common. And since they affect classroom performance, it's easy to see how they can be confused with ADHD. About 25 percent of children with ADHD also have a learning disability.[14] Like ADHD, learning disabilities do occur in families and are more common in boys, but the exact neurochemical connections between them are unclear.

The most common learning disabilities in ADHD children affect speech and language, memory, organization, and fine motor coordination. The actual manifestations of these disabilities vary from child to child. Common difficulties include dyslexia (confusing letters and words in text) and hand-eye coordination problems (for example, poor handwriting).

Sometimes a learning disability is difficult to diagnose because the child is bright enough to compensate for the weakness. It's not unusual, for example, for dyslexia to go unnoticed until adolescence or even adulthood.

Testing for a specific learning disability can usually be done within a school system by a school pschologist or a learning disabilities specialist. Sometimes the testing psychologist in an ADHD assessment will also test for learning disabilities. This might be done, for instance, when test scores or observations during the psychological evaluation lead to the suspicion that a learning disability is an important factor. Frequently psychologists suspect that a learning problem is present when they find a discrepancy between the IQ score as measured on the WISC-III and the score on an achievement test like the Wide Range Achievement Test—Revised. At other times, a psychologist may not be skilled in testing for learning problems and will refer the individual for further testing to an educational psychologist or an educational specialist.

Symptoms of learning disability can include:

• Poor comprehension of verbal and written material

• Poor recall of facts

• Difficulties with spatial relationships (confusing left and right directions)

• Difficulties with sequencing problems

• Specific difficulties with math, spelling, and reading

In most cases learning disabilities, which often are confused with ADHD, can be treated with a high degree of success. But before you make any treatment decisions, you should find out if further testing is required to confirm the new diagnosis, then ask the assessment team for resources to learn more about the disorder and obtaining treatment. Your child's teacher or counselor may also have valuable insights to offer on your child's learning ability.

CHAPTER SIX

How to Treat ADHD

*O*nce the assessment is completed and the presence of ADHD has been established, you'll receive some recommendations for treatment. Of the available ADHD therapies, the medicinal approach—specifically with Ritalin—is by far the most popular.

Medication is easy to administer, and it's fast-acting. It is also effective: even when used alone, it is helpful for up to 70 percent of children and an untold number of adults.[1]

You can therefore understand why Ritalin has the reputation of being a magic pill.

But the idea that one pill will fix the problem is short-sighted.

Most professionals who treat ADHD recommend a

multipronged treatment approach, combining medication and psychotherapy. Numerous studies support this approach, notably a 1992 study of twenty-four ADHD boys that concluded that the combination of behavior therapy and Ritalin had a greater positive effect on their behavior than Ritalin alone.[2] Arthur Anastopoulos and George DuPaul, writing in a 1991 edition of the *Journal of Learning Disabilities*,[3] reported that reviews of clinical studies of ADHD treatment indicated that the disorder requires multiple treatment methods that must be applied over the long term if they are to have any impact on the behavior of ADHD children.

These findings are not surprising when, if you are an adult with ADHD, you consider how far the ramifications of the disorder reach into your life. ADHD affects your physical, social, educational, and professional well-being.[4] Its symptoms can keep you up at night, alienate you from friends and family, cause learning difficulties, and hamper your career. Controlling the symptoms with medication and without maintenance, support, and retraining is like having a diabetic rely entirely on insulin and pay no mind to diet or exercise. In the case of ADHD, medication plays a critical role in controlling symptoms such as impulsivity and hyperactivity, but other therapies need to be utilized to prevent long-term complications such as isolation and aggression.

Steve Ogg was diagnosed with ADHD as an adult. When he started dealing with the disorder, he also started turning his life around. In a relatively short period of time he flourished professionally and his relationship with his wife and children improved enormously. Steve gives Ritalin credit for giving him the motivation to take control, but subsequent psychotherapy gets at least as much recognition.

The optimal multimodal treatment program should involve two or more of the following therapies:

• Medication

• Psychological interventions

• Educational interventions

• Supportive interventions

Let's see what each of these approaches contributes to the process of treatment.

Medication

Medications designed to adjust the imbalances of the brain's neurotransmitters can have a dramatic effect on ADHD. When they work, ADHD sufferers quickly show an increased ability to pay attention, concentrate, control impulses, and control hyperactivity.[5] No other treatment can produce such significant improvements in such a relatively short period of time—often as soon as the first time a person takes it.[6]

Chapters 7, 8, and 9 discuss medications in detail, but let us note here that two chief categories of drugs are prescribed for ADHD. *Psychostimulants* are the most commonly used medications. They include Ritalin (methylphenidate), Dexedrine (dextroamphetamine), Adderall (dextroamphetamine/amphetamine sulfate), and Cylert (pemoline).[7] Some young people with mild forms of ADHD may require medication for only a few years, or until they are able to develop strategies to cope with the symptoms.

Antidepressants have also been used with some success with ADHD children. Tofranil (imipramine), Norpramin (desipramine), Prozac (fluoxetine),[8] and Wellbutrin (bupropion) are helpful in dealing with ADHD accompanied by such problems as anxiety or depression. Because they're associated with more side effects and are generally less effective than stimulants, however, antidepressants are usually used only when stimulant medication doesn't work.[9]

When you see dramatic improvement in ADHD behaviors after medication treatment has begun, you might be tempted to believe that you've solved the problem. But again it's important to remember that medications control the symptoms of ADHD only temporarily. They can't help you or your child feel better about yourself or cope with problems more effectively. That's where other therapies come in.

Psychological Interventions

Psychotherapy can be enormously beneficial for ADHD children and adults, especially those who have low self-esteem and a somewhat distorted self-image. A supportive, trusting relationship with someone outside the family is often valuable in helping them develop a more positive sense of who they are. Psychotherapy is usually offered in individual, group, or family sessions.

For your ADHD child, your assessment team might suggest a specific approach to psychotherapy, such as behavior modification or social skills intervention, to help change troubling behavior patterns. Parent training classes and family therapy sessions can also teach you special techniques that will improve your relationship with your child and help you motivate positive behaviors. Even if you've raised other children with no problem, a child with ADHD can present challenges that exhaust your ordinary discipline techniques.

How psychotherapy can help you or your child is discussed more fully in Chapter 10.

Educational Interventions

Since ADHD children face so many unique challenges in school, educational interventions can make it possible for them to have a better chance for success. Tutoring and computer training can contribute to the treatment process by enhancing learning ability and decreasing classroom frustration for ADHD children and teens.[10] Special education classes can be beneficial for ADHD students, especially if they can't function well in a regular classroom.

In Chapter 12 more detailed information will be given about educational interventions and how you can decide if you or your child will need such services.

Supportive Interventions

Many, if not most, adults with ADHD, as well as parents of children with the disorder, will need support and help in coping with the everyday difficulties associated with ADHD. Locally sponsored parenting classes and individual and family therapy are good places to get extra insight and information; ADHD support groups can also help to address the social problems the disorder presents. In Chapter 10 you will learn more about how to find a support group in your area.

Nonstandard Treatment Approaches

As you research ADHD treatments—through reading books and magazine articles, talking to friends, or searching for more information on the Internet—you'll probably run into some "remedies" that aren't addressed in this chapter. *Diet therapy,* especially the Feingold method mentioned in Chapter 3, which advocates abstinence from refined sugars and food additives, is chief among them. Over the past thirty years researchers have made countless attempts to confirm the efficacy of diet therapy, but few studies have supported it.[11] Some ADHD sufferers, however, do report that cutting out sugar seems to help curb the symptoms.

"James Story," 19, for example, has taken Ritalin for several years. He says it helps him, but he also claims that the sugar-free food regimen he has followed since grade school makes him feel "focused and less hyper. Maybe it wasn't the sugar thing," he says. "Maybe it was just the practice I got at being disciplined. But I know my ADHD wasn't as bad."

Establishing healthier eating habits does require a certain degree of discipline and concentration. When you and your child are pursuing a course of action that brings you closer together and requires personal discipline, it may well have at least an indirect effect on the ADHD symptoms.

Sensory integration therapy is a treatment that is gaining in popularity for the remediation of motor and academic problems.[12] Many individuals with ADHD seem to have sensory integration dysfunction, which means an inability to derive useful information from sensory experiences. The sensory integration approach seeks to encourage the nervous system to process and integrate sensory input in organized and meaningful ways.

Other supposed ADHD "cures" include *EEG biofeedback therapy* (electrical therapy used to "train" the brain to control certain involuntary functions, like attention span) and *vitamin therapies*.[13] Pycnogenol, an antioxidant compound derived from the bark of the French maritime pine tree, is also included among these "cures." But so far, no medical or psychological study has shown them to be effective as a treatment for ADHD.[14]

The bottom line is that an alternative treatment—if approved by your physician, of course—that seems to help may be worth a try, but only in combination with therapies that are proven to be effective. And so far, the only treatment that scientific studies support is the multipronged approach that combines medication with psychological, educational, and supportive therapies.[15]

A final word of caution: Beware of "ADHD doctors" or "cures" advertised in magazines, on television, or on the Internet. Reputable services can't be provided via mail order, and they never require a check or money order "for more information."

CHAPTER SEVEN

Ritalin:
The Facts

*I*n the majority of ADHD treatment programs, when medication is a part of the therapeutic equation, nearly 90 percent of the time that medication is Ritalin.[1]

If you or your child begins taking it, you'll have lots of company.

Let's look at the reasons why Ritalin is the single most popular approach to ADHD treatment.

The Benefits of Ritalin

RITALIN IS HIGHLY EFFECTIVE.

Since the 1950s doctors and psychologists have been using Ritalin as a treatment for hyperactivity and

ADHD. No medication has since even come close to matching its effectiveness. Investigations and studies done at numerous universities have shown that Ritalin can reduce activity levels in seriously hyperactive children and substantially improve attentiveness in at least 70 percent of children with ADHD.[2]

To cite just one example, a carefully controlled study done at Lehigh University in Bethlehem, Pennsylvania, in 1993 compares both treated and untreated ADHD children with non-ADHD children, in the classroom, based on teachers' ratings of behavior. Neither the teachers nor the ADHD students themselves knew if the daily doses they were receiving were Ritalin or a placebo. The study found that the ADHD children who took Ritalin were virtually indistinguishable from the non-ADHD children in their attentiveness and academic performance.[3]

In another study comparing ADHD children on and off Ritalin, William Pelham and his associates at Western Psychiatric Institute and Clinic in Pittsburgh showed that the drug could even affect their baseball playing. Since baseball tends to be a slow game (especially for hyperactive individuals), Pelham wanted to know if ADHD children could meet its demands— paying attention, using judgment, and keeping track of the status of the game—if they took Ritalin. Reporting in the *Journal of Consulting and Clinical Psychology* in 1990, Pelham and his colleagues reported that Ritalin indeed had a positive effect on children's ability to focus on the baseball game and thus optimize their athletic performance.[4]

The key word here is *optimize*. Ritalin's impact can be immediate, dramatic, and miraculous, but it isn't long-term or far-reaching unless it's bolstered by other therapies in a multimodal treatment program.

RITALIN HAS AN EXCELLENT SAFETY PROFILE.

Two generations of use and hundreds of studies suggest that Ritalin is a comparatively safe drug and that it does not lead to serious side effects.

A typical study is the one done in 1993 at Columbia University in New York, which confirmed that Ritalin not only rarely produces significant long-term side effects, but when side effects do occur, they completely reverse when the medication is discontinued.[5] By now the safety of Ritalin has been demonstrated so many times that little, if any, research is currently being performed to confirm it.

As Dr. Paul Wender, director of the ADHD clinic at the University of Utah School of Medicine, writes in his book *The Hyperactive Child, Adolescent, and Adult*, "Ritalin and other stimulants are the most effective and safest medicines available in the treatment of ADHD children."[6]

RITALIN CAN PROVIDE THE CORNERSTONE FOR A SUCCESSFUL MULTIMODAL TREATMENT PROGRAM.

"The most consistent single component of a multidimensional approach is stimulant medication," says Dr. Michael Lechner, an ADHD specialist at the Hurley

Medical Center in Flint, Michigan. Most experts would agree.[7]

James Swanson, Ph.D., who directs a school in California for students with ADHD, says Ritalin can be "miraculous and phenomenal," even though the goal of his school is to teach students to manage their symptoms and eventually wean them from medication.[8]

Because of its effects on the neurotransmitters of the brain, Ritalin can:

• Increase attention span and the ability to absorb and retain information.

• Reduce fidgetiness or hyperactive behavior, so more tasks can be accomplished in less time.

• Reduce impulsive behaviors and aggressive tendencies, so social interactions with friends and family members are improved.

• Improve the ability to focus, so that greater benefits can be derived from other treatments, such as psychotherapy.

The importance of combining other therapies with Ritalin cannot be overstated. As Betty Osman of the White Plains Hospital Medical Center in White Plains, New York, puts it, "The young person should know that medication will not solve all his problems."[9] Jane E. Fried, at the Columbia University College of Physicians and Surgeons, makes the point that because children with ADHD are a diverse lot whose conditions have various causes and symptoms, "it is not surprising that a combination of medication and psychotherapy is more effective than either one alone."[10]

The Drawbacks of Ritalin

RITALIN ISN'T ALWAYS EFFECTIVE.

In some cases Ritalin just doesn't work. No one knows exactly why some people are unresponsive, and no one can predict if you or your child will be in that group.[11]

Many patients have a difficult time accepting this fact. And some, hoping for a miracle, see one even when it's not there. As Dr. Swanson says, "The expectation of the medicine can affect how people think it's working."

In most cases Ritalin works immediately, but it should be tried for four to six weeks (assuming there are no side effects) before a decision as to its efficacy is made. Too often anxious parents, children, and adults give up before they have given Ritalin a reasonable chance.

RITALIN HAS SIDE EFFECTS.

All medications have side effects, and stimulant medications are no exception. These are the most common physical disturbances associated with Ritalin.

Loss of appetite

Your child on Ritalin may say he's not hungry, or he may seem to be eating less. Children on Ritalin often have poor appetites, which is most apparent immediately after taking the pill.[12] These children will typically eat very small breakfasts and lunches but large dinners. Research has shown, however, that calorie counts during a twenty-four-hour period are approximately equivalent in the child both on and off medication.

Some children seem to experience an increase in appetite while they are on Ritalin. One reason may be that before taking the medication, the child would not sit still long enough to eat, but with the medication he is able to sit at the table calmly and finish a meal.

Treatment or prevention: If your child's eating habits change or weight loss occurs, do not hesitate to call your doctor. The doctor may want to weigh and measure him on a regular basis and, if necessary, adjust the dosage. If your child loses more than three percent of total body weight in the first three months of therapy, consideration should be given to lowering the dosage or changing the medication.[13]

This common side effect usually goes away as the youngster becomes adjusted to the medication. But some children do experience an ongoing loss of appetite that often worries parents. Dr. Fried suggests that loss of appetite occurs chiefly at lunchtime. To avoid this, she recommends that the morning Ritalin dose be administered after breakfast, that the afternoon pill be given after lunch, and that children have an opportunity for an after-school snack.[14]

Insomnia

Several studies have shown that ADHD children have a higher likelihood of sleeping problems than non-ADHD children. Russell Barkley reported in *Psychiatric Annals* in 1991 that as many as 56 percent of ADHD children (compared with 23 percent of non-ADHD kids) take a long time to fall asleep. In addition, Dr. Barkley reported, up to 39 percent of ADHD children may show problems with frequent night waking.[15] Almost all children have difficulty falling asleep or awaken early when they begin taking Ritalin. Within a few weeks, however, the body appears to adjust and the children sleep normally.[16]

Treatment or prevention: If your child still has problems falling asleep after a week or so, you might consider Benadryl or a "natural" compound called melatonin before bed. But first consult your doctor. Your doctor can recommend an appropriate dosage of either Benadryl or melatonin. Benadryl is available at any drugstore, and melatonin is available at most health food stores.

Many parents also find it helpful to place a fan in the child's bedroom. This "white noise" muffles other distracting sounds and helps the child fall asleep faster. Your doctor may also try to reduce or eliminate your child's afternoon dose of Ritalin. If sleep problems continue, your doctor may suggest changing medications.

Gastrointestinal disturbance

A gastrointestinal disturbance could be anything from a stomachache to nausea with vomiting or diarrhea. If your child is younger, she may say she simply doesn't "feel good."[17] Usually these symptoms go away within one week, especially after the medication has been adjusted to the appropriate level.[18] If your child is vomiting or in serious pain, call your doctor immediately.

Treatment or prevention: Taking medication after a meal, or after a snack in between meals usually resolves the problem. A small dosage of Maalox after taking the Ritalin pill may help. If complaints of stomachaches continue beyond one week, your physician may advise a different medication.[19]

Headaches

Headaches occur in some children either while they are on Ritalin or while it is wearing off. The headaches are not often severe but are persistent. Sometimes they can be an indication that the Ritalin dosage is too high.[20] If the headaches persist for more than a week, get progressively worse, or interfere with the daily routine, contact your doctor.

Treatment or prevention: Your doctor might suggest treating the headaches with acetaminophen (Tylenol) or ibuprofen (Motrin or Advil). If they persist, it's likely that the medication will have to be changed.[21]

Increase in heart rate or blood pressure

Many people who begin treatment with a stimulant medication experience elevations in their resting heart rate and blood pressure. Children may describe these symptoms as a feeling that their heart is racing or pounding. The symptoms subside as the body adjusts to the drug.[22]

A review of Ritalin studies in 1992 by Dr. Daniel J. Safer indicated significant elevations in heart rate at the beginning of stimulant treatment, but when treatment was continued, the increase was minor. Long-term stimulant therapy resulted in no unusual symptoms.[23]

Treatment and prevention: Your doctor should routinely monitor your child's heart rate and blood pressure before starting therapy and every two or three months thereafter. If the blood pressure and heart rate remain elevated for more than three weeks, the dosage should be altered or the medication changed.

Rebound

Rebound is associated with Ritalin's rapid exit from the body. It usually happens at the end of the day, when the last dose wears off. During this time the child or adult may be prone to crying or emotional outbursts. Because of the quick mood swing, rebound is also referred to as the "Ritalin roller coaster."

Treatment or prevention: If the rebound is debilitating or interferes with the child's or the family's daily routine, ask your physician about trying a very small dose of Ritalin at the end of the day. Such a minute amount won't correct attention and hyperactivity problems but may alleviate the rebound.[24] Sustained-release Ritalin, which provides a steady flow of stimulant, is another potential solution to the problem. This may smooth out the mood fluctuations. Some doctors prescribe a combination of short-acting and slow-release Ritalin to maximize effectiveness and minimize rebound.

If your child is having this problem, try making evenings as stress-free as possible.

Miscellaneous and Rare Effects

Other side effects of Ritalin include irritability, nervousness, and dry mouth. These symptoms are usually temporary and are typically caused by an improper dosage. Again, report them to your doctor.[25]

Hair loss, skin rashes, joint pain, and dizziness are also listed as side effects of Ritalin. These nonspecific reactions can, however, occur with any number of medications—Tylenol, for example, can cause a rash—so their significance relative to Ritalin is debatable. The minute risk of developing one of these side effects should not preclude a trial of Ritalin. If any of these problems should occur, contact your physician.[26]

Very rarely, Ritalin therapy may be associated with serious complications. They include:

Seizures
Seizures or convulsions are sudden, uncontrollable contractions of muscles caused by abnormal electrical

discharges from the brain. Normally the brain is able to control its electrical activity, but if it is stressed or sensitized, there may be an overload, leading to a seizure. Ritalin doesn't directly cause seizures, but in some rare instances it can hinder the brain's ability to control its own electrical activity, and seizures may result. Seizures should always be reported immediately to your doctor. Single transient seizures are not associated with any long-term neurological damage.[27]

Treatment or prevention: If seizures do occur, the medication should be stopped immediately and the doctor contacted. The seizure problem usually resolves itself once the medication is stopped. Ritalin therapy should be permanently discontinued.[28]

Bone marrow suppression

The bone marrow produces all of the blood cells. When it is hindered from this job—or suppressed— the supply of blood cells is diminished, and serious illness, like anemia or infection, can result. There is no way to predict the probability of this rare side effect of Ritalin.[29]

Treatment or prevention: Before starting you or your child on Ritalin, and yearly thereafter, your doctor will want to analyze a blood sample. This sample provides your doctor with a baseline reading of your blood with which future blood samples can be compared. If it is later found that the bone marrow is not producing blood appropriately, Ritalin should be discontinued. In the case of patients with blood disorders or kidney disease, extra care should be taken to monitor blood and kidney functions.

Psychosis

Psychosis is a severe mental condition characterized by hallucinations or delusions. There have been newspaper reports that Ritalin has caused psychosis,[30] while some supposedly authoritative sources also indicate that this is a potential side effect.[31]

Dr. Arthur Robin has used Ritalin in his practice for two decades. "I've never had a patient who has been medically harmed by Ritalin," says the chief of psychology at Children's Hospital of Michigan. "No suicide, no psychosis, none of that."[32]

Other experts agree. Dr. Martin Baren, writing in *Contemporary Pediatrics*, explains, "There are reports of a psychotic-like syndrome produced in very small numbers of children taking Ritalin and other stimulants. We are not certain whether the syndrome is a unique event or whether it occurs when children with some type of underlying psychotic process are placed on the medication. The numbers are very small, and the symptoms disappear when the medication is stopped."[33]

In our review of several thousand research reports and studies, we found only two journal articles describing psychotic reactions in just two children.[34]

Like many other medications, however, Ritalin can exacerbate preexisting psychosis. If you have a family history of schizophrenia, manic-depressive disorder,

or paranoia, or have psychotic tendencies, the drug
should be avoided.

Other Fears About Ritalin

IS IT A COPOUT, A "QUICK FIX" FOR
BEHAVIORAL PROBLEMS?

Parents who put their children on Ritalin often encounter criticism from their friends. Those who don't
understand that ADHD is an organic disorder tend to
think of parents who turn to Ritalin as unable to control their children. For parents who tend to blame
themselves—most of us—such criticisms are influential.

   People criticize Ritalin because they have heard
stories about its abuse and misuse. They may have
seen, or heard about, children who are poorly monitored after being placed on Ritalin therapy. These
misconceptions and unfortunate exceptions provide
ammunition for the anti-Ritalin forces. Peter Breggin,
M.D., is one of the most outspoken Ritalin critics
in the United States. In his book *Toxic Psychiatry*, he
refers to hyperactivity as "the invention of a disease."[35]
And in his latest book *Talking Back to Ritalin: What
Doctors Don't Tell You About Stimulants for Children*,
Breggin charges that the FDA and the NIMH have
failed to tell the public the truth about Ritalin's potential danger.[36] You're likely to run across at least one
person who shares his views.

"People sneer at you and give you dirty looks when you tell them you're giving your kid a pill that helps him get through the day," says "Jan Lee." Even though her son, Matt, did well on Ritalin from the very beginning, she found it hard not to let the criticisms get to her.

"But I realized my antagonists hadn't been through the bad grades, the temper tantrums, the assessment," she says. "The voice inside my head, telling me it's okay, is the voice of experience."

IS IT ADDICTIVE?

For people with ADHD, Ritalin only normalizes brain function. It does not give them a perceivable high. Therefore they do not crave the drug.[37]

Ritalin is a strong amphetamine, however, and can give people without ADHD a feeling of invincibility and hyperalertness. Some people may find this feeling appealing and become addicted to its stimulant effects.

In a 1995 study conducted on both humans and baboons, generic Ritalin was tested to see if in fact it had some of the same potentials for a "high" that cocaine has. The study, reported in the *Archives of General Psychiatry*, noted that although there has never been any evidence that Ritalin produces a "high" and subsequent addiction when taken orally, it was run to see what would happen if the drug was taken intravenously. The result was that any "high" rapidly disappeared. The authors concluded that this quick disappearance of any "high" would serve as a limiting factor against frequent self-administration of Ritalin.[38]

CAN IT LEAD TO SUBSTANCE ABUSE?

Some experts believe that ADHD children who are *not* treated with Ritalin may be more likely later to go on to substance abuse.[39] Children with ADHD do have higher rates of drug addiction than the general population, mainly because of their impulsive, risk-taking behaviors and, in some children, overlapping aggressive tendencies.[40] In addition, a growing body of research indicates that ADHD children and adolescents turn to drugs and alcohol as an attempt to self-medicate, in order to feel more calm and relaxed.[41] When a person is properly treated with Ritalin, however, he becomes less impulsive and is better able to consider the long-term consequences of his actions. Therefore he is less likely to abuse drugs, alcohol, and tobacco.

"The research has not demonstrated that giving kids methylphenidate for ADHD increases the risk for drug abuse in later life," says Dr. John Werry, a prominent ADHD expert in New Zealand. "No evidence at all."[42]

And no, prolonged use does not result in increased dosage requirements.[43]

CAN IT STUNT GROWTH?

Studies performed by D. J. Safer and R. Allen and their associates at Johns Hopkins University Medical

School in the early 1970s suggested that long-term use of Ritalin resulted in a decreased adult height.[44] But numerous subsequent studies have failed to duplicate this result.[45] A 1996 study reported in the *Journal of the American Academy of Child and Adolescent Psychiatry*, which examined nearly 125 ADHD children and a similar number of control subjects who did not have ADHD, found that any height deficits in ADHD children disappear by late adolescence. No weight deficits were detected in ADHD children and teens. The authors, echoing other recent research studies, concluded that children with ADHD may have temporary deficits in height but that their height normalizes by the late teenage years. These researchers also concluded that this height deficit is more likely associated with ADHD, not Ritalin usage.[46]

In summary, then, no research in the past twenty years has proven that Ritalin stunts growth.[47]

CAN IT CAUSE CANCER?

A recent study stated that Ritalin causes liver cancer in laboratory mice,[48] but these results have been criticized by the Food and Drug Administration (FDA) and other experts.[49] The study, conducted by the National Toxicology Program (a branch of the National Institutes of Health) and reported in the journal *Toxicology* in 1995, administered various doses of Ritalin to rats and mice (many up to thirty times what is normal for children or adults to receive) for periods lasting from two weeks to two years. Under the conditions of the experiment, no evidence of cancer was found in the rats that received doses of Ritalin over two years. But some indication of cancer was found in the livers of the mice in the shorter trial periods.

When the study was reported by the Associated Press in January 1996,[50] it provoked a wide range of reactions from experts, even within the National Institutes of Health. Alan Zametkin, a specialist in ADHD at the National Institute of Mental Health, stated, "This study was done now because no previous carcinogenity studies have been done. . . . How is it we have drugs in the market, approved by the FDA, with no previous carcinogenicity studies done? I find it startling."[51] Ritalin was approved by the FDA in 1955.

In an FDA press release, spokesman Don McLearn explained that the "signal" that Ritalin might produce cancer in this study was "weak"; that mouse liver is known to be very susceptible to the development of tumors; and that the kind of liver tumor found in mice is "extremely rare in people."[52] The significance of these results to humans is unknown, but previous studies of Ritalin have shown it to have a low risk of causing cancer.[53] The FDA has labeled it as having a low cancer risk but suggests further study.[54]

Taking Ritalin

DOSAGES

Ritalin is always prescribed in pill form and is always intended to be taken orally. Initially, your doctor will probably figure your child's total daily dose at 0.2 milligrams per 10 pounds of your child's body weight (50 pounds × 0.2 = 10 milligrams). The pills come in 5, 10, and 20 milligram doses and are usually taken twice a day. Five milligrams, twice a day, is a common starting dosage for children.[55]

After a few weeks of monitoring the medication's effects and side effects, a physician may decide to raise or lower the initial dose. Most physicians will rely heavily on your input—as a patient or as a parent—to help them make adjustment decisions (as discussed in Chapter 8).

Some physicians have found success with Ritalin doses of up to 0.5 milligrams per pound.[56] For a 50 pound child, the usual daily dose would range from 15 to 20 milligrams but could go as high as 60 milligrams. The eventual dose of Ritalin is based only on your child's response and not on age, weight, or degree of symptoms. A first-grader may need 60 milligrams a day, while a high school senior may need only 5 milligrams a day. The dosages may be just as variable in adults.[57]

DOSAGE TIMING

The first daily dose of Ritalin is usually taken just before breakfast in the morning. Whether it's taken before, during, or after breakfast makes little difference in terms of how it is absorbed or when it becomes effective. Generally Ritalin becomes effective thirty to sixty minutes after ingestion.[58] You may want to time your child's dosage so that it coincides with the beginning of the school day. Peak effectiveness occurs within two to three hours after it is first taken; that effectiveness begins to decrease after three hours and usually has worn off entirely by about six hours after ingestion. The second pill should be taken right around noon, to compensate for the lag time between the two doses. By the time the first dose wears off, the second dose will have become effective. Timing is particularly critical for children who need to sustain their attention and concentration through the school day.

Without a third dose, Ritalin generally clears the system by early evening and therefore doesn't disturb sleep. A third dose given around three or four P.M. can help with homework and home behavior. If you feel that a third dose is necessary and it doesn't affect sleep habits, there's usually no reason to avoid it.[59]

What You Need to Report to the Doctor

So that your doctor can make an accurate assessment of your or your child's *progress* on Ritalin, you should report the following information:

• Any side effects (especially weight loss and sleep disturbance)

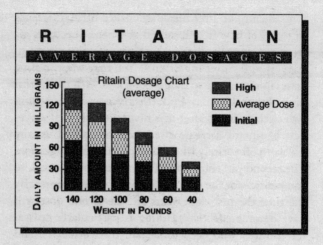

• Changes (positive or negative) in school or professional performance. For example, have grades improved?

• Changes (positive or negative) at home. For example, is your child arguing more with siblings?

• Changes in mood. For example, does your child seem teary or depressed in the evening?

• Attitude about Ritalin. For example, how does your child feel about taking Ritalin at school?

• Changes in social relationships. For example, is your child making new friends?

• Anything at all you don't understand about the drug or the dosage.

A word of caution: It is possible for both children and adults to overdose on Ritalin.

Ritalin should be taken in the dosage prescribed, by mouth. Increases in dosage, or snorting or injecting the drug, can result in tragic consequences, even death.[60] Signs of overdose include vomiting, agitation, tremors, seizures, increased heart rate, sweating, and confusion. Any person who is suspected of having a drug overdose should be taken to a hospital emergency room immediately. There the person will likely have his stomach pumped, be placed on intravenous fluids, and be admitted to the hospital.

When handled with care, Ritalin is a safe and effective drug. The best way to prevent any potential problems is to follow your physician's exact prescription instructions.

Different Types of Ritalin

Ritalin is available in two varieties. Short-acting Ritalin comes in 5 milligram, 10 milligram, and 20 milligram tablets, while Ritalin-SR (sustained release or slow-acting Ritalin), is available in 20 milligram tablets. In addition, a generic form, methylphenidate hydrochloride, is also available. Theoretically there is no difference between the three types of medication, but many patients report that the generic form seems less effective.[61]

Pharmaceutical regulations require that generic drugs be at least 75 percent as effective as brand-name medications. This does not mean that generic drugs are of lower quality—there's a possibility that they just might be weaker. So if a patient switches from brand-name Ritalin to the generic form, many physicians will increase the generic dose to compensate.

There have also been conflicting reports about the effectiveness of the longer-lasting form, Ritalin-SR. One study, published in 1989 in the *Journal of the American Academy of Child and Adolescent Psychiatry*, showed that while the sustained-release form of Ritalin lasts longer, it never quite reaches the same level of effectiveness as an identical dosage of short-acting Ritalin.[62] To overcome this effect, physicians will prescribe both types for some patients: they will give their concentration a quick boost in the morning with short-acting Ritalin, and then maintain the drug's effects throughout the day with the sustained-release pills.[63] There are also indications that sleep disturbances increase in patients taking sustained-release Ritalin, which may pose another drawback to its use.[64]

Some children have trouble swallowing Ritalin pills even though they are small. A practice session with M&Ms might help your child get the knack. Ideally, Ritalin pills shouldn't be chewed. If your child continues to have trouble, try disguising the pills in a spoonful of applesauce or ice cream.

COST

Prices vary, but as a rule brand-name Ritalin runs about 25 percent higher than generic. Most prescriptions will range from $40 to $70 per month.

Many medical insurance plans offer reimbursement for the pills or include them in prescription coverages. You should call your insurance company or pharmacist to find out about your coverage.

Ritalin as a Controlled Medication

Ritalin is a Schedule II controlled substance that is available only by handwritten prescription. Its distribution is tightly controlled by the Drug Enforcement Administration (DEA), and it is dispensed in strict accordance with state regulations.[65] Prescriptions must be filled within seventy-two hours, and no refills are permitted.

Drugs are placed on a schedule based on their abuse potential. Recently CHADD (Children and Adults with Attention Deficit Disorder) petitioned the DEA to reclassify Ritalin from a tightly controlled Schedule II medication—the same category as opium, morphine, and cocaine—to a less tightly controlled Schedule III medication.[66] Since some studies, such as the one comparing Ritalin to cocaine,[67] have shown that its abuse potential is fairly low, reclassification would simplify the prescription process by allowing the physician to phone in prescriptions and by permitting refills.

Eliminating some of the bureaucracy involved in the manufacture and distribution of Ritalin may help lower the price, since Schedule III medications are not subject to strict manufacturer quotas that can result in shortages for patients.

What to Expect from Your Doctor

A responsible physician will carefully monitor the dosages and effects of Ritalin. Before you or your child begins treatment, your doctor should get a clear picture of the patient's health by ordering a battery of blood tests, including a hemoglobin level, platelet count, liver function, thyroid function, and lead level. The doctor should then repeat the blood tests every year to make sure the medication is not causing any subtle long-term side effects.

Once treatment has begun, your physician should schedule regular follow-up visits to ensure that the medication is given in proper amounts and that no serious or surprising side effects are developing. The visits should be monthly at first; once the dosage is stabilized, they can be scheduled biannually. Monthly appointments early in treatment are opportunities to answer questions that have arisen, clear up any misperceptions or confusion (on either the parent's or child's part), and encourage the family to undertake other interventions that will assist in management of the ADHD symptoms.

During your follow-up visits, the doctor should

also carefully measure your child's height, weight, blood pressure, and heart rate. Alterations in these numbers can be the first indication of potential side effects. If your physician does not monitor these basic statistics on a regular basis—or simply prescribes medication without requesting follow-up visits—you may want to consider a change.[68]

Ruling Out Ritalin

Some people simply shouldn't use Ritalin. They include the following categories.

Young children

Although some experts, such as Russell Barkley,[69] suggest that Ritalin treatment is neither justified nor effective with preschoolers, virtually no studies on preschoolers and the use of Ritalin exist. Both Barkley and Lydia Fusetti (and her associates)[70] contend that medical treatment of children below the age of four may lead to more severe side effects or may prove less effective. In young children distinguishing between normally active behavior, oppositional behavior, and ADHD presents a difficult diagnostic problem, as has been pointed out by Susan Campbell, who has studied ADHD in preschoolers.[71]

Patients taking other medications

Certain medications may potentially interact in negative ways with Ritalin. These include antihistamines, antidepressants, anticoagulants, and anticonvulsants.[72] The hypertension medication guanethidine may be less effective if used with Ritalin.[73] By contrast, the anticoagulant Coumadin, the anticonvulsants phenobarbital and Dilantin, and the antidepressants Tofranil and Norpramin are broken down more slowly when taken with Ritalin, which makes their effects more potent. Therefore the dosages must be decreased.

To avoid drug interactions, notify your physician and your pharmacist about any medication—prescription or other—that you or your child may be taking.

Patients with a history of tics

If you have a family history of tics, it should raise legitimate questions about using Ritalin. Recently researchers have investigated the connection between tics and Ritalin use. Prescribing Ritalin should be done only after serious consideration (as discussed in Chapter 5).[74]

Women who are pregnant or breast-feeding

No current research is available about the potential hazards of using Ritalin if you're pregnant or breast-feeding.[75] Based on the evidence of other similar drugs, however, it is very likely that small amounts of Ritalin would be passed through the placenta or the breast milk to the infant. It is likely therefore that, unless the mother has a significant need for the medication, it should be stopped during pregnancy and breast-feeding.

People with certain physical conditions

If you or your child has high blood pressure, seizure disorders, severe anxiety, or glaucoma, the patient shouldn't take Ritalin. Previous allergic reactions to stimulant medications are another obvious reason to avoid the drug.

Once you're comfortable with Ritalin on a pharmaceutical level, you'll want to consider the Ritalin do's and don'ts presented in Chapter 8.

CHAPTER EIGHT

Ritalin
Do's and Don'ts

These do's and don'ts are a quick reference guide addressing some of the most common issues in Ritalin treatment.

DO HAVE PATIENCE WHEN IT COMES TO WORKING OUT THE DOSAGE.

Sometimes it takes several weeks to get the Ritalin dosage right.[1] For safety's sake, your doctor will begin with a relatively low dose and increase it in small increments until the benefits are maximized and the side effects minimized.[2] There's no way to predict how much Ritalin you or your child will need. Some adults do just fine with two 10 milligram doses a day, while some young children function best with two 40 milligram doses.

If your doctor puts your child on an initial low dose and it doesn't work, don't throw in the towel. It's understandable if you're timid about increasing the dosage; you've probably heard some scary things about the drug. Be patient. Let your doctor gradually increase the dosage until it is effective.

Along the way there may be side effects to work through. Occasional stomachaches, headaches, slight weight loss, and loss of appetite could stay with your child for just a few days or several weeks.[3] Side effects often disappear when the dosage is optimal, but these problems must be evaluated on a case-by-case basis. You may have to make a decision: Do the side effects of Ritalin outweigh its benefits?

DON'T ASSESS EFFECTIVENESS BY YOURSELF.

Assessing the effects of Ritalin—like assessing for ADHD in the first place—should be a group effort.

Combining the insights of parents, teachers, physicians, and psychologists is the most useful way to assess the drug's success. An overview of home behavior, classroom participation, physical response, and psychological adjustment offers an objective answer to your most pressing question: Is Ritalin working for my child? Because Ritalin brings about such a dramatic improvement for a majority of children, the answer to this question is usually obvious. Children who experience subtle changes are more difficult to gauge, and for them, a team evaluation is especially helpful.

A team evaluation offers other benefits as well. You or your child with ADHD has an increased potential for long-term psychological, emotional, and behavioral problems.[4] Ritalin alone won't improve them, and your assessment team can help you decide what kind of adjunct therapies you may need.

DON'T TAKE IT UPON YOURSELF TO ADJUST THE DOSAGE.

If your child is having a particularly stressful day, he might actually ask you for more Ritalin. This isn't because he's craving it or having withdrawal symptoms but because he's learned, from listening to you and the doctor and everyone else involved, that Ritalin helps him function better. He's also experienced improved control of his attention, focus, and hyperactivity. Who can blame him for liking it?

Don't give in to his request. Ritalin dosages should never be altered without your physician's order.[5] Too much of the drug might indeed be dangerous.[6]

Adults very often are tempted to experiment with or modify their medication, but the same rule applies: To avoid any harmful side effects, leave dosage adjustments up to your physician.

DON'T TAKE DRUG HOLIDAYS OR
DISCONTINUE RITALIN FOR A WEEKEND.

ADHD is a physical disorder that is with you all the time. Diabetics don't stop taking insulin just because it's Sunday. Likewise, children and adults need relief from the symptoms of ADHD all the time.

The demands of everyday life are just as important as the demands of the classroom or the workplace. Evenings and weekends are filled with a variety of activities, including everything from soccer games to catechism. Enhancing skills only from eight A.M. until three P.M. Monday through Friday is unfair to parents and children.

Taking the medication intermittently also gives children a distorted view of its purpose. They should view the Ritalin as a part of their lives and not as a quick fix for troublesome situations.

Some physicians reduce the dosage or eliminate Ritalin use during long vacations or during the summer, but only if the child's personal and academic demands are going to be significantly diminished.[7]

DO TRY TO MAINTAIN A POSITIVE ATTITUDE.

A little animosity goes a long way. Younger children, especially, are quite sensitive to their parents' feelings. If they sense that you're apprehensive about the pills, then they might become apprehensive as well.

Usually parents and adults worry about what

they've heard about Ritalin. Check your sources. Are the claims you're fretting about scientifically proven? You should discuss your concerns with your doctor. If this fails to assure you, visit a support group meeting.

Teenagers in particular sometimes resist taking Ritalin—or simply stop taking it—usually for reasons that have nothing to do with the drug's effects.[8] Drug taking becomes one more battleground in the adolescent power struggle and the effort to assert greater personal autonomy. In other words, rebelling against their Ritalin regimen is one way teenagers can feel like they're more in control of their own lives. Maria Gallardo, for example, resents every yellow pill she puts in her mouth. "I don't want someone to tell me what I need to do," the thirteen-year-old says, "especially a grown-up."

As a compromise, Maria made a deal with herself and her parents. "I'm going to quit it for a while when I'm sixteen. If things go okay, then I'll stay off. If things don't go okay, I'll get back on."

She takes her Ritalin twice a day nonetheless, since "it does help me with schoolwork." In fact, she is now an honor student, though she used to struggle for C's.

DON'T BE SURPRISED IF RITALIN SEEMS TO CAUSE CHANGES IN PERSONALITY, BUT REPORT THESE CHANGES TO YOUR DOCTOR.

In most cases the behavioral changes brought about by Ritalin are quite welcome. Without Ritalin, your child might be extremely hyperactive and therefore unable to make friends. He might also be suffering in school and driving everyone crazy at home. On the other hand, hyperactivity may make your child outgoing and bubbly, traits that may be especially endearing to you. A few children do, in fact, become less spontaneous when they're treated with the drug.[9] "Sometimes the child's very nature is intrinsically tied up with hyperactivity, particularly in the preadolescent," says Arthur Robin, Ph.D., chief of psychology at Children's Hospital of Michigan and a noted ADHD expert. "This is something that has to be handled with utmost sensitivity."[10]

If your child appears even remotely dazed or unusually passive, or exhibits any new aggressive or bizarre behavior, it could be an indication that he has been overmedicated. But if you or your child is one of the few on whom Ritalin has an emotionally "flattening" effect, even at an optimal dosage, you may have to make a decision: Do the drug's positive effects outweigh its effects on personality?

DON'T EXPECT AN OVERNIGHT MIRACLE.

Ritalin can have a dramatic and immediate effect on the primary symptoms of ADHD, but it will take time before these improvements begin to have an impact. ADHD's symptoms took a while to pervade your child's life, eventually damaging everything from schoolwork to friendships. Undoing the damage caused by the primary symptoms can be achieved only when

Ritalin therapy is combined with at least one other type of treatment, such as psychotherapy or family counseling.

Taking care of the primary symptoms is the easy part. Taking care of the secondary problems— behavioral, self-esteem, and academic problems—is more difficult and time-consuming.

And finally, one last piece of advice:

DO CONSIDER OTHER MEDICATIONS IF RITALIN DOESN'T WORK.

Don't give up on all medications if the use of Ritalin has proven to be unsuccessful.[11] Various other medications could have a beneficial effect on your child, which will be discussed in the next chapter.

CHAPTER NINE

Other Medications for ADHD

Although Ritalin is the most commonly prescribed medication for ADHD, it is not the only drug, nor is it necessarily the right one for you or your child.[1]

ADHD is a complex disorder, with many different presentations. One person with ADHD may experience hyperactivity, while another may have difficulties with impulsivity. Each will have a unique response to medication.

Even when Ritalin does work, it may need some help. As we have seen, people with ADHD also may suffer from a related disorder, such as depression or anxiety, which could require an additional medication. The medications used to treat ADHD are divided into three general categories: stimulants, antidepressants, and miscellaneous drugs.[2]

NINE OTHER MEDICATIONS FOR ADHD

Adderal (destroamphetamine): A short-acting stimulant medication

Cylert (pemoline): A long-acting stimulant medication

Dexedrine (dextroamphetimine): A short-acting stimulant medication

Norpramin (desipramine): An antidepressant medication

Prozac (fluoxetine): An antidepressant medication

Tofranil (imipramine): An antidepressant medication

Wellbutrin (bupropion): An antidepressant medication

Catapres (clonidine): A high blood pressure medication

Haldol (haloperidol): A tranquilizer used in the treatment of tics

---

Stimulants

Stimulant medications affect those with ADHD in a way radically different from the way they affect people without it. If you were asked: What type of medication does someone who can't sit still need? You'd probably guess Valium or something else that would calm the person down. But for ADHD sufferers, that guess would be wrong. What calms them down is stimulant medications. In people with ADHD the levels of two neurotransmitters in the areas of the brain that control attention are abnormal. Stimulant medications normalize these levels by stimulating the parts of the brain that govern focusing and processing information and therefore control the symptoms of ADHD.

Different stimulant medications seem to affect different specific areas of the brain. For example, Cylert will increase a certain neurotransmitter's activity in one area, while Ritalin will increase it in another. These variations explain why certain people have a better response or fewer side effects with a particular medication. Since we can't determine which part of the brain is affected in any given individual, finding the best treatment often involves some trial and error.

All stimulant medications have a few things in common.[3] First, they seem to have little long-term addiction potential for people with ADHD. Since stimulants normalize brain function in people with ADHD, they do not give them a perceivable high, and this tends not to foster drug cravings.

Second, the eventual dosage of each stimulant medication is based on a person's response to the drug and not on his or her age, weight, or degree of symptoms.[4] You can see a kindergartner on 60 milligrams of Ritalin per day and a high schooler on only 5 milligrams per day, both with good control of their ADHD. Usually people start out on small dosages, which are increased until their behavior is controlled and the side effects are minimized.

Third, although each of the stimulants may have its own particular side effects, the two most common adverse reactions are sleep disturbance and poor appetite.[5] A small percentage of people on a stimulant medication will complain of headaches, which may not be severe but may be persistent. Usually headaches can be treated with acetaminophen (Tylenol) or ibuprofen (Motrin or Advil) without changing stimulant medications or dosages. Of course, these and any other unusual effects of a stimulant should be reported to the prescribing physician.

Each of the stimulant medications has its own advantages and disadvantages. Although Ritalin is typically the first medication to be tried, other stimulants may be more effective, have fewer side effects, or be better suited to your or your child's lifestyle.

The most commonly prescribed stimulant medications (besides Ritalin) are Adderall, Cylert, and Dexedrine.

ADDERALL (DEXTROAMPHETAMINE/ AMPHETAMINE SULFATE)

Background

Adderall is one of the newest stimulants used to treat ADHD. It's a combination of four types of amphetamines plus dextroamphetamine. An effective alternative to Ritalin, it has the advantage of being administered in a single dose per day. Adderall is available as 10 and 20 milligram tablets.

Advantages
• The tablets are double-scored. This allows them to be broken easily for more flexible and precise dosing. Ritalin is not scored.

• Adderall is a slower-releasing medication and therefore can be taken only once per day, rather than in several doses, as Ritalin is.

• It is specifically approved for use in children as young as four.[6] (But children younger than five should not be medicated for symptoms of ADHD.)

Disadvantages
• Similar to Ritalin[7]

Side effects
Rapid heart rate, dizziness, increased blood pressure, restlessness, euphoria, poor appetite, insomnia, tremors, tics, impotence, abdominal pain, and dry mouth

Other uses
Adderall is also used to treat narcolepsy, a type of sleeping disorder in which a person spontaneously falls asleep.[8]

Most likely ADHD patient
A younger child who has not responded well to Ritalin, or any individual who only wants to take one daily

dose of medication. Since teenagers are often resistant to taking medication, they may agree more readily to taking one dose.

Cylert (pemoline)

Background

Cylert is the newest of the stimulant medications. When it was originally introduced, it was heralded as the only drug a person would ever need for the treatment of ADHD.[9] Although it has failed to meet this high expectation, it does provide an effective alternative to Ritalin for many people. Overall, it is used in about three percent of all ADHD children on medication, with a slightly higher percentage of teens and adults.[10]

Cylert is available as 18.75 milligram, 37.5 milligram, and 75 milligram tablets, and as a 37.5 milligram chewable tablet.

Advantages

• Cylert is a long-acting medication, so unlike Ritalin, it is taken only once per day. This schedule is advantageous for children who are reluctant to take medication during the day at school or for busy, forgetful parents, as well as for adult ADHD patients.

• A chewable tablet is practical for children who are unable to swallow pills.

Disadvantages

• Unlike Ritalin, Cylert's effects are not immediate. It takes weeks to build up therapeutic levels in the bloodstream. Until this stabilization of blood levels occurs, parents may not notice any changes in their child's behavior. Ritalin, by contrast, causes an immediate, often dramatic response.

• Cylert must be taken continuously in order to maintain therapeutic levels in the bloodstream. If a patient misses more than three days on Cylert, it may take a week to build back to effective levels.[11]

• Because Cylert is processed by the liver slowly, it takes weeks to fully disappear from the body. Therefore physicians often suggest tapering off the medication rather than stopping it abruptly. Tapering is unnecessary with Ritalin.

• Cylert is not specifically approved for use in children less than six years old, although some physicians will use it in this age group.[12]

• There have been reports of liver damage following long-term use of Cylert.[13]

Side effects

Rapid heart rate, sleepiness, dizziness, tics, restlessness, tremors, poor appetite, insomnia, abdominal pain, and nausea

Other uses
None

Most likely ADHD patient
A teenager who wants to take one dose per day, a younger child who needs a chewable tablet, or a child or adult who doesn't respond to Ritalin.

DEXEDRINE (DEXTROAMPHETAMINE SULFATE)

Background
Dexedrine is one of the oldest medications used to treat ADHD and is used by five percent of children with ADHD.[14] Dexedrine is available as a 5 milligram tablet, or as 5 milligram, 10 milligram, and 15 milligram capsules (or Spansule or slow-release form).

Advantages
• Dexedrine has a rapid onset of action. Usually symptoms begin to improve within a half hour of taking the dose, and the effects last approximately five hours.

• The slow-release form allows the child to take pills only one or two times a day, thus eliminating the need for that potentially embarrassing lunchtime visit to the school nurse.

• It is specifically approved for use in children as young as four.[15]

• It is slightly less expensive than Ritalin.

Disadvantages
• Dexedrine has relatively more side effects (such as appetite suppression and sleep disturbance) than Ritalin and therefore is usually a second-choice drug.

• It is known as speed in its street form and is abused by large numbers of drug addicts.[16] Although abuse is rarely a problem with ADHD children, physicians are often hesitant to prescribe it because of the stigma.

• Acidic foods such as orange and pineapple juice interfere with the absorption of Dexedrine. Patients should avoid acidic foods within one or two hours of taking the pills.[17]

Side effects
Insomnia, appetite suppression, rapid heart rate, dizziness, increased blood pressure, restlessness, tremors, tics, abdominal pain, and dry mouth

Other uses
It also is used to treat narcolepsy and as an appetite suppressant.[18]

Most likely ADHD patient
A child age four to six.[19]

Antidepressants

People are often confused by the term *antidepressant*. True depression is more than a feeling of sadness. Like ADHD, it is a chronic medical disorder, caused by a neurotransmitter imbalance in the brain. Antidepressant medication can improve the symptoms of depression by correcting the levels of the neurotransmitters norepinephrine and dopamine in the brain. Antidepressants also are used effectively for a variety of conditions, including bedwetting, eating disorders, drug addiction, and ADHD.

To understand how antidepressants and stimulants differ in action, consider this analogy. First, picture your brain as a sink and the water in the sink as the neurotransmitters. The sink should normally be full, but in those with ADHD it is only, say, half full. In order to fill the sink to the correct level, you can do one of two things—turn up the water or plug up the drain.

Plugging the sink increases the water level by interfering with the outlet, which is what an antidepressant does—it maintains the levels of neurotransmitters by interfering with their breakdown. Turning on the faucet keeps the sink full by providing a constant stream of water, which is what a stimulant medication does—it maintains normal levels of neurotransmitters by promoting their release.

The end results are similar, but the biggest problem with antidepressants is that they are less effective on ADHD than stimulants.[20] Plugging the drain is never quite as efficient as turning up the water. Therefore antidepressants are used only if stimulant medications fail or cause severe side effects. The dosage of antidepressants is adjusted similarly to that of stimulants: Patients are started on a low dose first for a few weeks, while being carefully monitored for response and side effects. The initial dosage is slowly increased until good control of ADHD symptoms is achieved, with minimal side effects.[21]

Although antidepressants are less effective, they have some very distinct advantages over stimulants. First of all they are not addictive.[22] If a person who is not depressed or does not have ADHD takes an antidepressant, he is basically unaffected. But if that person takes a stimulant, he or she will definitely feel anxious, hyperalert, and agitated. For some teens, these feelings are desirable. Kids with ADHD have been known to sell, increase the dosage of, or even smoke their stimulant medications. If a child has had problems with drug abuse in the past, the doctor may elect to remove the temptation and prescribe an antidepressant.

Second, antidepressants enhance sleep and do not affect appetite as much as some stimulants do. Appetite suppression and insomnia are two of the most commonly reported side effects of stimulants, Ritalin in particular.

Third, antidepressants positively affect mood. Researchers have shown that approximately 50 percent of ADHD children have some type of emotional disorder, such as low self-esteem, emotional instability, and anxiety.[23] It is not often clear whether these symptoms of depression are a result of ADHD or simply exist in combination with it. (It is known that depression is very common in children. For example, up to 30 percent of teenagers will be clinically depressed at times during their adolescent years.)[24] Since they reduce the symptoms of both depression and ADHD at the same time, antidepressant medications can be especially helpful in certain cases. Many physicians have begun prescribing combinations of stimulants and antidepressants with good results.[25] But because of the complex effects that multiple medications have on the body, this practice should be limited only to those who have failed single drug treatments.

The biggest problem with antidepressants is that they are less effective on ADHD than stimulant medications in general. They also have a slower onset of action. The major side effect of nearly all antidepressant medications is sleepiness, which can be a problem for obvious reasons.

The most commonly used antidepressants are Norpramin, Prozac, Tofranil, and Wellbutrin.

NORPRAMIN (DESIPRAMINE)

Background
Norpramin is very similar to Tofranil but has fewer side effects. It does not cause tics and has a slightly lower risk of heart problems.[26] It is available as 10

milligram, 25 milligram, 50 milligram, 75 milligram, 100 milligram, and 150 milligram tablets. It can be an effective alternative for those who fail to respond to stimulants.

Advantages
• Norpramin can be taken only once a day, thus eliminating a lunchtime dose.

Disadvantages
• Norpramin can cause significant drowsiness, which can be debilitating.[27]

Side effects
Dizziness, increased or decreased blood pressure, rapid heart rate, disorientation, confusion, hallucinations, numbness, incoordination, seizures, blurred vision, breast enlargement, flushing, urinary retention, abdominal pain, and dry mouth

Other uses
It is mainly used to treat depression.

Most likely ADHD patient
A child or adult with ADHD and depression who did not respond to Ritalin alone.

PROZAC (FLUOXETINE)

Background

Despite the constant bombardment of negative publicity about Prozac, it remains the most widely prescribed adult antidepressant in the United States, with researchers constantly discovering new uses for it.[28] Patients with impotence, phobias, drug addiction, bulimia, and other conditions (some not yet specifically approved for Prozac treatment by the FDA) have been helped by Prozac. It is gaining favor among pediatricians for the treatment of depression in children who also have ADHD.[29] The early results of studies about Prozac indicate that it may be the most effective and best tolerated of the antidepressants for children who are depressed and in addition have persistent ADHD symptoms.[30] Although Prozac by itself is not frequently used to treat ADHD, in combination with Ritalin it can be effective. Prozac is available as 10 milligram and 20 milligram capsules.

Advantages

• Prozac is given only once per day.

• It has fewer side effects than other antidepressants.

• It does not require routine monitoring via electrocardiograms (EKGs) or blood work.

Disadvantages

• A great deal of controversy surrounds Prozac, which may make you reluctant to use it. The sensationalized stories, reported in the media, of an increased risk of violent or suicidal behavior have so far not been substantiated by researchers. It is likely that violent behavior and suicidal thoughts existed in these patients before they were on Prozac.

• It is very expensive and costs much more than other antidepressants.

• It can precipitate seizures and should therefore be used with caution in patients with any history of them.[31]

Side effects

Dizziness, sleepiness, weakness, chills, rapid heart rate, abnormal dreams, disorientation, confusion, hallucinations, abdominal pain, dry skin, sensitivity to light, joint pain, breast pain, and urinary retention

Other uses

It is used to treat depression and obsessive-compulsive disorder.

Most likely ADHD patient

A child or adult with depression and ADHD who is not responding to Ritalin or another psychostimulant.

TOFRANIL (IMIPRAMINE)

Background

Tofranil is the most widely used antidepressant for ADHD.[32] It is viewed as a moderately effective alternative to stimulant medications. Some researchers have reported it to be 80 percent successful in children who have some depressive symptoms along with ADHD and who initially did not respond to stimulants.[33] It is available as 10 milligram, 25 milligram, and 50 milligram tablets, which are small and easy to swallow.

Advantages

• Tofranil is most often taken once a day, usually just before bedtime. This eliminates the need for a dose to be given at school.

• Interestingly, it is also very effective for the treatment of nighttime bed-wetting, since one of its side effects is urinary retention. For a select group of children with ADHD and bed-wetting, it may be an effective alternative.[34]

Disadvantages

• Tofranil can exacerbate tics.[35] It should therefore be avoided in children with prior tics or a family history of tics. If tics are observed, the medication should be stopped immediately.

• It takes several days to build up effective blood levels and so does not produce the immediate response that Ritalin does. Because it requires this steady blood level in order to be effective, it must be taken continuously.

• It may increase the risk of heart problems such as arrhythmias. The risk of developing a heart problem is increased in patients with a family history of heart disease. Doctors will often order an EKG to be done before a patient starts Tofranil if it is believed there is any risk.[36]

• It is safe when taken in the proper dosage but can be fatal in an overdose, which can occur with as few as ten tablets. You must be ultravigilant about keeping it away from small children. If a teenager or an adult expresses any suicidal thoughts, the pills should be taken away immediately.

• Because of Tofranil's potential long-term effects on the liver and heart, the doctor may require a yearly blood test and EKG.[37]

Side effects
Sleepiness, dizziness, increased or decreased blood pressure, heart arrhythmias, tics, disorientation, confusion, hallucinations, numbness, incoordination, seizures, blurred vision, breast enlargement, urinary retention, abdominal pain, and dry mouth

Other uses
It is mainly used to treat depression and bed-wetting.

Most likely ADHD patient

A child with ADHD and bed-wetting, or a child or adult with ADHD and symptoms of depression who does not respond to Ritalin alone.

Wellbutrin (bupropion)

Background

Wellbutrin is a new kind of antidepressant that acts on different neurotransmitter pathways from other drugs. Since its introduction to the arsenal of drugs used to fight ADHD, it has had favorable results with relatively few side effects.[38] It is available as 75 milligram and 100 milligram tablets and is usually taken three times a day.

Advantages

Similar to the other antidepressants.

Disadvantages

• Wellbutrin is associated with an increased risk of seizures and should therefore be used with caution in people with a prior history of them.[39]

Side effects

Headaches, dizziness, dry skin, tremors, sleepiness, confusion, hallucinations, seizures, urinary retention, weight loss, abdominal pain, and dry mouth

Other uses
It is mainly used to treat depression.

Most likely ADHD patient
A child or adult with ADHD and depression who does not respond to Ritalin alone.

Miscellaneous Medications

Several medications outside the antidepressant and stimulant categories are effective in reducing the symptoms of ADHD. Because these medications are often much less effective than either stimulants or antidepressants, they are most often relegated to third-choice drugs. They may be useful to those with particular symptoms or severe reactions to other drugs. Two of the more commonly used medications in this category are Catapres and Haldol.

CATAPRES (CLONIDINE)

Background
Catapres is a commonly prescribed antihypertensive or blood-pressure-lowering medication, which is also the most widely used of the third-choice drugs for treating ADHD.[40] The exact mechanisms by which Catapres controls the symptoms of ADHD are not fully understood. Catapres is available as 0.1 milligram, 0.2 milligram, and 0.3 milligram tablets.

Advantages

• Catapres is especially helpful in the treatment of ADHD sufferers with tics. It was actually found to be an effective treatment for tics before it was discovered to be a treatment for ADHD.[41]

• It can benefit the subgroup of ADHD children with very high activity levels, which may not be controlled by Ritalin. Catapres often is able to improve extreme hyperactivity and reduce the resultant aggressive and rebellious behavior.[42]

Disadvantages

• Because Catapres is primarily an antihypertensive medication, children and adults taking it can have significantly lowered blood pressure.[43] They should be monitored closely and the medication adjusted as needed.

• The most common side effect of Catapres is drowsiness, which can be significant and impair schoolwork. A significant number of children placed on Catapres continue to have excessive sleepiness despite lowering the dosage and must discontinue it.

• Catapres must be discontinued slowly to avoid a rapid increase in blood pressure.

Side effects
Dry mouth, dry eyes, low blood pressure, weakness, high or low heart rate, rash, dizziness, headache, fatigue, and sleepiness

Other uses
It is used to treat high blood pressure, Tourette's syndrome, migraine headaches, and withdrawal from drugs, alcohol, and tobacco.

Most likely ADHD patient
A child or adult with ADHD and tics or with ADHD who is very hyperactive and does not respond well to Ritalin alone; a child or adult with ADHD and high blood pressure.

HALDOL (HALOPERIDOL)

Background
Haldol is a tranquilizer used in the treatment of psychotic disorders and Tourette's syndrome. The strong connection between Tourette's and ADHD has been acknowledged for years. It is believed that, depending on which particular symptoms are more prevalent, certain individuals might be diagnosed as having either Tourette's or ADHD. Haldol is one of the most effective treatments for Tourette's syndrome, although it may block the effectiveness of methylphenidate when the two drugs are used in combination with each other.[44] It is available as 0.5 milligram, 1 milligram,

2 milligram, 5 milligram, 10 milligram, and 20 milligram tablets.

Advantages:
• Haldol has been found to be an effective medication for children with tics,[45] but it does little to control the symptoms of ADHD.

Disadvantages
• Haldol can cause severe drowsiness. The drowsiness can be debilitating, and therefore the drug is used only in special circumstances.

Side effects
Drowsiness, high heart rate, low blood pressure, jaundice, dizziness, muscle spasms, depression, and hallucinations

Other uses
It is used to treat psychotic disorders (such as schizophrenia) and Tourette's syndrome.

Most likely ADHD patient
A child or adult with Tourette's syndrome or psychotic symptoms and ADHD; a child or adult with psychotic symptoms and ADHD.

Several other experimental medications have recently been reported to be helpful in treating ADHD. Some of these include Pondimin (fenfluramine, an appetite suppressant), Effexor (venlafaxine, an antidepressant), and Tenex (guanfacine, an antihypertensive). None of the initial studies on these medications show them to be nearly as effective and safe as Ritalin.[46] Although research is continuing, there does not appear to be any new magic pill on the horizon.

CHAPTER TEN

Psychological Treatment, Parent Training, and Support Groups

*M*edication is *never* enough to treat ADHD.

Even the most miraculous Ritalin response does not obviate the need for other supporting therapies. The National Institute of Mental Health[1] and the results of dozens of studies maintain that the most significant and long-lasting gains in the treatment of ADHD come with a combination of psychological treatment, behavioral therapy, and practical support, along with medication.[2]

The prospect of such a comprehensive treatment program can seem intimidating, but for children and adults with ADHD and their families, professional support can offer tremendous relief.

If you're the parent of a child with ADHD, you know how complicated life can be. ADHD children sometimes get in trouble at school and often lose friends because of their quick tempers and impulsive behaviors. They may spend hours trying to cope with homework and then forget to take it to school or lose it in their backpack. You struggle with the idea that maybe your child is lazy or unmotivated. Your attempts to mediate between your ADHD child and siblings and friends are often unsuccessful. Your attempts to run interference seem endless. Your attempts to remind, reassure, and relax your child are rejected or just plain ineffective. You get frustrated, you get tired, and you get angry.

If you're an adult with ADHD, life can often seem overwhelming. You may be disorganized and unable to focus. You have a difficult time finishing things, whether it's a load of laundry or a stack of paperwork. Your temper may flare at the slightest provocation, and as a result, your social and personal life suffers.

Almost every child and adult with ADHD, whether treated or not, will suffer some psychological consequences at some point in his or her life. The degree of these problems is often related to when treatment is initiated. The earlier treatment for ADHD begins, the better the outcome.[3]

Many types of psychological treatment are available, and among them is an approach that is right for you, your child, and your family. The members of your assessment team should be able to recommend qualified professionals who can provide the treatment you prefer. This treatment should include at least one type of psychotherapy.

Psychotherapy

Psychotherapy, a term that covers various types of counseling and psychological treatment, is a process that helps people resolve personal problems and make changes by talking with a trained professional.

There are two prerequisites for successful psychotherapy:

• You cannot approach the process with an attitude. Being open to the ideas and suggestions of an objective party is essential.

• You must be comfortable with your therapist.

A little research may be necessary to choose the right psychotherapist. Anyone can claim to be a psychotherapist, but most states have laws and certification procedures for persons qualified to provide psychological treatment. Usually, you will select one of the following professionals.[4]

• **Psychiatrist:** A psychiatrist is a physician holding an M.D. or D.O. degree, which means four years of medical school, a state medical license, and a four-year supervised psychiatric experience called a residency. Psychiatrists can conduct psychotherapy and can prescribe medication.

• **Psychologist:** A psychologist will have a Ph.D., Ed.D., Psy.D., M.A., or M.S. degree, plus several years of supervised work experience, along with a state license. Psychologists are qualified to do therapy as well as to administer psychological tests.

• **Social Worker:** Most social workers will have a M.S.W. degree. This degree often includes supervised counseling training, and social workers certified by the Academy of Certified Social Workers (ACSW) have completed at least two years of supervised clinical experience. Clinical social workers are able to do psychotherapy and family counseling.

• **Clinical Counselor:** A clinical counselor has at least a master's degree in counseling with certification by the National Board for Certified Counselors (CCMHC) and two years of supervised counseling or psychotherapy experience. Certified clinical counselors (CCMHC) are qualified to do psychotherapy and are sometimes trained to do substance abuse counseling.

Every psychotherapist will have advanced training in certain specialty areas. It's important that the one you select have experience in treating ADHD children and their families.

Approaches to Psychotherapy

There are many approaches to psychotherapy, from psychoanalytic psychotherapy to behavioral therapy.

Most therapists will use one particular treatment approach but vary their methods on a case-by-case basis. Therapies based on psychoanalytic principles require a long-term process that could take place over several years, while more contemporary psychotherapies, like cognitive-behavioral treatment, are short-term or brief. The most popular approaches today include:

COGNITIVE CHANGE

Cognitive therapies are based on the premise that changes in values, beliefs, or attitudes will lead to changes in behavior. In cognitive-oriented therapy, the therapist focuses on distortions and fallacies in thinking. The core of the therapy is to support the individual in correcting these thinking errors. Your ADHD child, for example, may feel inadequate. A cognitive therapist can help him correct this distortion.

BEHAVIOR MODIFICATION

Behavioral therapies are based on the premise that changes in behavior will produce corresponding changes in beliefs and assumptions. In general, behavioral therapy rests on the idea that behavior that is reinforced is strengthened, while behavior that is ignored or punished decreases in strength or is phased out. A behavior therapy program might reward your ADHD child, for example, whenever he stops to think about the consequences of his behavior instead of acting in an impulsive manner.

SOCIAL SKILLS TRAINING

Social skills training approaches center on teaching new behaviors that lead to more satisfying social relationships. Typically social skills training involves helping ADHD children learn to be more assertive communicators and to handle their anger in more effective ways. It also teaches them how to resolve conflict without resorting to aggressive behaviors.

Therapy Type: Individual, Family, or Group

Psychotherapies can also be distinguished by the role of the therapist and the client in the counseling sessions. In some approaches the individual seeks counseling, and therapy takes place in a one-to-one setting. In others several clients are treated at once in a group setting, using the group as a therapeutic medium. Still other approaches direct the therapy at the total family system and sometimes include members of the extended family. The most popular therapies—or at least elements of them—can be used with individual, group, or family approaches.

Individual, group, and family therapies are available at private mental health clinics, social service agencies, and community mental health centers, and from psychotherapists in private practice. Costs range from $50 to $200 per session. Lower fees, or fees based on ability to pay, are usually offered by social service organizations and community mental health centers. Usually group therapy is less expensive than individual therapy. Your health insurance may cover all or part of the fee.

INDIVIDUAL PSYCHOTHERAPY

Individual therapy offers a supportive, trusting relationship with an adult outside the family, which is often valuable in helping youngsters view themselves, their efforts, their behavior, their peer relationships, and their goals in more objective and positive ways.

In individual therapy children (and adults as well) with ADHD can talk about upsetting thoughts and feelings as well as their self-defeating behavior patterns. The goal is to change the patient's behavior and show him or her alternative means of handling emotions. As they talk, the therapist tries to help the patient understand how to change. In addition, psychotherapy can help a person change his self-concept from that of an inadequate underachiever to that of a more competent and consistent individual. Psychotherapy can also address such issues as self-control, the management of anxiety, and social skills deficits.

Children and teens with social skill deficits frequently have poor control over their emotions and have difficulty resolving problems in nonviolent and non-aggressive ways. In treating ADHD children and teens, some therapists concentrate on particular social skill deficits and teach young people techniques for overcoming their areas of weakness.

For example, eight-year-old "Jason Askins" was frequently in trouble at home and at school for fighting and for aggressively attacking peers who made him mad. In therapy Jason was taught to "stop and think," to control his behavior and respond in more appropriate ways with peers. After three months of therapy his parents found that the weekly calls from the principal had virtually ended. In addition to stopping and thinking, Jason was taught to take deep breaths when he started to get angry and to think about his new conflict resolution skills before he acted in an aggressive way.

Thirty-five-year-old "Brenda Parton" was very disorganized both at work and at home. She had started college years before but had quit in frustration because she couldn't concentrate on homework. After being diagnosed as having ADHD, she entered psychotherapy. While medication helped, in her weekly individual therapy sessions she tackled such issues as self-esteem, organization, impulsivity, and self-doubt. Within twelve sessions Brenda was more self-confident and engaged in less self-blame. Learning how to deal with her self-doubt, she improved her ability to handle her own expectations at home and at the office. She began to make plans to return to college with renewed enthusiasm and with new confidence in her abilities.

Individual therapy with ADHD children and teens can be effective, but usually it's alternated with group or family sessions. Adults with ADHD may opt for family or conjoint treatment but are less likely to do so than children and teens.[5]

Who can benefit

ADHD children and adults who recognize the problems related to their disorder and are willing to address them.

FAMILY THERAPY

Living with an ADHD child or adolescent can be rough on everyone in the house—brothers, sisters, and especially parents. As a parent, you may experience a range of emotions including shame, embarrassment, fear, anger, and guilt over your child's behavior. You may feel that you're neglecting the needs of your spouse and your other children because of the challenges of handling your ADHD child. Your own support network—friends and extended family—may become strained, either because you have your hands full supervising your child or because your child's behavior makes it difficult to be around friends or family.

"Randy Phillips" was an absolute terror before his ADHD was treated. As long as his mother, Susan, could remember, life with Randy was a constant string of tantrums.

"And he had Superman syndrome," she says. "He thought he could leap over small buildings. He just lost all common sense."

At first friends and family seemed to sympathize with Susan and her husband, "Sean." But after a year or so, they started to turn away and criticize. "One teacher told me, 'I think you need to love him more,'" Susan says. "Our whole family was just barely hanging together by a thread."

It's easy to see how ADHD can stress even the strongest marriage. You and your spouse may disagree over discipline (or the use of medication), or you may have difficulty finding time for each other because you are exhausted by your efforts to care for your impulsive, hyperactive, or distractable youngster. Family therapy can be very useful in addressing these conflicts.[8]

Although there are various types of family therapy—just as there are different types of group therapy—all have the same goals of strengthening the family as a system and improving the ability of all family members to communicate better and solve problems more effectively.

Who can benefit

Families experiencing communication problems as a result of ADHD.

"I think counseling can be more helpful for parents than kids sometimes," says "Elaine Dunbar." Four of her five sons have been diagnosed with ADHD. "There's a grief reaction. There's a terrible guilt trip."

Elaine says family therapy has helped her tremendously. Her sons also are doing well. "My God, I nagged them incessantly before I knew what was wrong. And they're so forgiving. But you know, we never would have been able to air all this out alone."

GROUP THERAPY

Friends are very important to school-age children, but youngsters with ADHD almost always suffer problems in groups. Usually their difficulties derive, in part, from their poor ability to fully understand and use social cues, to control themselves, and to follow rules, as well as from their tendency to be competitive and aggressive. A group therapy approach often can address these problems better than individual therapy can, because as troubled interactions emerge, they can be corrected on the spot.

Various recent studies have examined the effectiveness of group therapy for ADHD children. James Lock, M.D., Ph.D., professor of psychiatry and behavioral sciences at Stanford University School of Medicine, reported in 1996 that groups that were developed to help with self-control and social skills could be very helpful in the overall treatment of ADHD children.[6]

William Pelham, an ADHD researcher at the Western Psychiatric Institute and Clinic in Pittsburgh, has shown in several studies that ADHD children in group therapy have improved classroom behavior and better academic performance as compared with ADHD children who are on medication alone.[7]

Who can benefit
Children and adolescents who aren't able to talk openly about their problems in individual therapy or who have problems in peer relationships. This could apply to adults as well, but there are generally fewer group therapy opportunities for adults.

Parent Training

Whether you get help in individual, group, or family therapy, learning new or improved parenting tools and discipline techniques will help you to better manage your ADHD child's behavior.[9] In fact, after medication, parent training is the second most common treatment approach to helping the ADHD child or adolescent. While individual or family therapy can show parents how to cope, parent training classes are specifically designed to teach them disciplinary and child management skills, often in a classroom atmosphere, with practice, rehearsal, and homework. Learning these skills in a group with other parents provides for valuable cosupport and interaction that rarely occurs in other types of treatment.

Some recent research even suggests that in many cases parent training is *required*—along with medication—to effectively treat ADHD youngsters.[10] Arthur Anastopoulos and his associates stated in the *Journal of Abnormal Child Psychology* in 1993 that their studies showed that parent training classes reduce parental stress, increase parental self-esteem, and reduce their child's ADHD symptoms.[11]

Parent training classes are available through mental health clinics, hospitals, schools, community education programs, and libraries, and as special seminars sponsored by ADHD support groups. These classes are often free or involve a minimal charge.

Who can benefit
Parents who need help learning new and effective discipline skills, or who are simply at their wit's end.

Support Groups

ADHD support groups such as Children and Adults with Attention Deficit Disorder (CHADD) are another valuable resource for ADHD children, adults, and their families. Support groups for parents of ADHD children have been growing rapidly in the past decade; led by CHADD's 32,000 members in six hundred chapters, they are now available in every state and large city in the United States.[12] Support groups are usually free.

Parents have been attracted to these support groups for the opportunity to share experiences as well as practical tips with others who have been on the front lines. Attending a support group could help you to meet other people who have experienced the same emotional difficulties, like guilt, that you may be experiencing. Or you may feel isolated; especially if you receive little support elsewhere and are feeling stressed out, an ADHD support group can be a lifeline. Additionally, support groups usually provide lectures, books, and handouts to help you keep up on the latest thinking in ADHD.

Jeannie Kime is in charge of a local group that meets monthly.

"It runs itself, really," she says. "I just sort of guide it out of ruts."

There are usually two dozen people or so in her group, who come to share their frustrations and successes, listen to knowledgeable speakers, exchange referrals to qualified specialists, and trade information about what works and what doesn't.

Jeannie's husband and son both have ADHD, and she finds she's able to field questions from adults with the disorder and from parents.

"We're not in the business of dispensing medical advice," Jeannie says. "But we'll help you find someone who can."

Many adults who have ADHD also find that

attending a support group leads to greater insight and understanding about themselves and the best ways to make sure treatment works.

In the Resources section of this book, you'll find a listing of national organizations that can help you find a support group in your area.

CHAPTER ELEVEN

Parenting the ADHD Child

Children with ADHD generally have behavior problems just as non-ADHD children do—only more so.

In fact, that's a pretty good way of describing the ADHD child; they are more so. If all children are active and sometimes overactive, the ADHD child is more so. If all children sometimes act without thinking, the ADHD child does it more so. And if most children have a short attention span sometimes, the ADHD child has one more so.

Put these three characteristics of ADHD children—hyperactivity, impulsivity, and distractibility—together, and you not only have a "more so" child, you very likely have one who gets into a little more trouble and is more difficult to parent.

Such a child can disrupt your home, put extra stress on your marriage, and, no matter how calm and stable you are by nature, make you appear—and feel— like anything but a calm and rational mom or dad. Many parents of ADHD children feel tremendous amounts of stress.[1]

The Stress of Raising an ADHD Child

"Kathleen Reilly," the mother of five-year-old "Mikey," a hyperactive boy always on the go and always "into everything," says she often felt like a "raving lunatic."

"I used to yell at Mikey, and he wouldn't pay any attention to me," Kathleen says, "so I'd yell louder. I found myself screaming at him in malls. Once I grabbed him like a crazy woman and started to shake him in a store, and another woman came along and told me she was going to call the police if I didn't calm down."

"Debby Ellis," the mother of eight-year-old "Krissy," who was diagnosed as ADHD at age six, be-came depressed at dealing with her daughter. "After a few hours together with her not listening to me and going from one thing to another," Debby says, "I'd lock myself in my room and cry. I was sleeping more, and I was starting to drink wine early in the afternoon in order to cope with our fights and arguments."

Many parents of ADHD children say the toughest part of coping is dealing with the energy, the disobedi-ence, and the oppositional behavior of their child. Because of the experiences of parents like Kathleen and Debby over the years, several research studies have looked at the stress that parents of ADHD youngsters experience.[2]

What these studies found may not surprise you. Mothers of seven-year-old ADHD children, for instance, seek treatment for personal problems much more often than mothers of non-ADHD seven-year-olds.[3] As expected, mothers of ADHD children of all ages report markedly higher levels of stress and depression than parents of children without ADHD.[4] Furthermore, parents of ADHD children suffer greater marital discord than do couples with non-ADHD children.[5]

The kinds of psychotherapy discussed in Chapter 10 can help you cope with an overwhelming complex of problems by reducing them to some more manageable goals. Here are four important ones:

1. Have reasonable expectations of your child.
2. Understand why ADHD children misbehave.
3. Create a successful home environment.
4. Take care of yourself.

Goal 1: Have Reasonable Expectations of Your Child

Asking a hyperactive child to sit still for a prolonged period of time is like asking him to change the color of his eyes. When you accept this fact, then you'll be able to begin to manage his problems effectively.

Modifying your image of your ADHD child doesn't mean you have to change your expectations of him. You can still have high expectations. The majority of children with ADHD are of at least average intelligence, and you can expect that your child will learn to behave in an acceptable manner and that she will have average or above average grades at school—in time. With the appropriate intervention, she can grow up to be well-adjusted and successful.

Goal 2: Understand Why ADHD Children Misbehave

Why do ADHD children misbehave?

The fact is that impulsive children do many things without thinking. When they are frustrated or provoked, they often react with anger and with no degree of thought. They explode in rage, or they throw the nearest toy. If they are teased by a sibling, they respond impulsively. No matter how many times you remind them, when they are calm and under control, not to hit or to throw footballs in the house, they react next time as if you'd never told them. Impulsive behavior is frequently aggressive, but not because the child has no feelings for others or has defects in his moral development. It's just that when he reacts quickly, sometimes his behavior seems angry and is aggressive.

The fact is, too, that distractible children simply forget what they are supposed to do. They get side-tracked by other things. Children sent to clean their room forget what they are there for and may end up playing a game or reading. It's not that they intend to disobey—they just get sidetracked when something else catches their attention.

The fact is, also, that hyperactive children are likely to lose interest in chores, tasks, reading, and homework. They get antsy and fidgety. They frequently engage in a lot of random behavior. When a young child or even an adolescent has a need to expend physical energy, sometimes he does whatever impulsively crosses his mind. It's not meant to annoy, bother, or even hurt you, it's just what the hyperactivity demands.

How you react to these behaviors can make a difference as to whether your child learns better self-control or continues to act in impulsive and out-of-control ways.

If you react to early temper tantrums and aggressive behavior with passivity and indulgence, her behavior will continue and may get worse. If you are overly strict and harsh, using punitive methods of control, you are likely to create even more serious behavior and management problems. Failing to discipline consistently will tend to lead to continued "misbehavior."

Goal 3: Create a Successful Home Environment

Granted, it's not easy to discipline perfectly and lovingly at all times. But as a first step toward dealing with your ADHD child, it will help to create a home and family environment that will support his learning to control his behaviors.

A successful home and family environment for your family as well as your ADHD child will provide two essential things. First, it will provide structure, and second, it will provide appropriate discipline.[6]

STRUCTURE

A well-defined structure within a family provides the rules, limits, and boundaries that help a child who has self-control problems know where his behavior must stop. A reliable structure involves the following:

• Making sure rules and limits are well defined

• Making expectations clear and explicit

• Giving rule and expectation reminders frequently

• Redirecting unacceptable behavior

• Providing close supervision and monitoring

• Making sure rules are fair and consistent

• Spelling out consequences for rule violations that are always the same and firmly applied

A good starting point for defining rules and limits is to establish fixed family routines. It has been shown in several different studies that ADHD children do best when they are provided with a structured daily schedule.[7] Otherwise, while doing homework, the ADHD child may only think, "I wonder what time dinner will be tonight?" If the child knows that dinner is at six o'clock every day, he is more likely to concentrate on the homework.

Take time each day to write and post a daily schedule, then stick to it. Place a check next to each item as it is completed. You may even go so far as to schedule exact menus, daily outfits, play activities, and travel times.

It's also important that you define your expectations and rules for your child. You should not define too many important rules, but you should certainly have a few that apply to the children in your family.

For instance, in the "Miller" family, "Tom Miller," father of nine-year-old "Ryan," expects his children to do well at school, be involved in sports, be respectful to adults, and do their assigned chores every day. Those have been the expectations in the family from the time "Timothy," Ryan's older brother, was a toddler.

The expectations and the rules need to be explained and made clear to the children, whether they have ADHD or not. Although Tom Miller talks about the rules often, to help Ryan, who has ADHD, Tom also wrote them on a chart and posted it on a bulletin board in the kitchen.

Even when the expectations and rules are discussed and posted, children with ADHD still need reminders. When Ryan goes outside to play with his friends, his father goes over the "outside rules." He does this by asking Ryan to tell him what the rules are.

"When you go to your friend's house," Tom Miller says, "what will you remember to do?"

"Be polite," Ryan begins to recite, "don't go to anyone else's house without coming home first and asking you, and . . ."

"And come home before dark," his father says, reminding Ryan of the rule that he has forgotten in the past.

Redirecting unacceptable behavior is important, too, and it can often be done in lieu of admonishing or punishing the child. When Tom finds Ryan throwing a baseball against the kitchen wall, he doesn't just yell at him. He gently guides him outside and shows him a constructive alternative—throwing the ball against the back of the garage. By doing this, Tom manages to keep the entire interaction positive.

To help a child who often doesn't think before acting, close supervision may be required. Keeping track of where the child is and what he's doing is necessary until the child learns better self-control. Tom will sometimes call the house where Ryan is playing just to see how things are going. When Ryan goes to a nearby school playground to play basketball, his father will stop by to "watch." He thinks it's important to let Ryan know he's checking up on him and that he will monitor where he is and what he's doing.

Once your expectations and rules are established, you need to enforce them in a consistent and firm manner, showing your child that his actions have definite consequences. That way, he can predict what kind of trouble he will be in if he disobeys.

When Ryan comes home after dark, his father is waiting for him, and Ryan knows he is in trouble. Sometimes Ryan gives excuses: "I didn't know it was this late," he says. Other times he says, "Davey's mother didn't tell me what time it was."

But his father doesn't buy into his excuses. "Ryan, you know what the rule is. You're to be home by dark. Now you will have to stay in the house tomorrow after school. No playing outside. I want you to learn that when there's a rule, it's your responsibility to follow it."

Giving your child this kind of consistent structure means he will have a better chance to learn to be responsible and conform to your expectations and rules.

APPROPRIATE DISCIPLINE

There's no question that disciplining a child with ADHD can be challenging. You may even have concluded, after trying all the discipline techniques you know, that "nothing works." Your frustration can often lead to inflicting progressively harsher punishments for misbehavior. To get your discipline approach back into focus, you will have to have a detailed plan that you can call to mind when you need it:

Praise and reward good behavior.

With a difficult ADHD child, it is easy to get into the No! No! No! mode. Too often parents of an ADHD child focus on all the things he's doing wrong and forget about the things he does right. If you want to increase those appropriate behaviors, you must praise them. Give more attention to your child when he's done something right than when he's done something wrong.

As a result of their underachievement, ADHD children frequently develop low self-esteem. Giving your child positive reinforcement in the form of praise or a tangible reward will build his self-worth, even as it encourages more positive and praiseworthy behavior.

Use effective commands.

Another habit many parents fall into is using ineffective or too frequent commands. Ineffective commands are those that begin with *don't* or *stop*. "Don't touch the TV." "Stop hitting your sister." "Don't yell in the house." "Stop running." *Don't* and *stop* commands are difficult for ADHD children to obey.

Other ineffective commands are those that are too vague ("Be good at the restaurant"), too complicated ("Get ready for bed. Brush your teeth, take a shower, pick up all your clothes on the floor of the closet, and be sure you go to the laundry room and bring up your clean underwear") or ask questions ("Would you like to clean Kitty's litter box?").

The most effective commands are specific, clear, simple, and direct, and they are "do" commands.[8] Here are some examples:

> "Bring me the book, please."
> "Please come inside the house."
> "I want you to brush your teeth."
> "Pet the dog this way, okay?"

Each of these commands is more likely to be followed, especially if you give the child praise and attention for compliance.

Ignore certain misbehavior.

When you try to handle every misbehavior and stop every objectionable behavior, you're going to end up giving a lot of ineffective commands. Also, you may find yourself yelling, nagging, or just feeling frustrated and exasperated all the time.

It is essential, therefore, to learn to ignore certain behaviors—minor, irritating, annoying, and attention-getting misbehaviors such as whining and tattling—obviously, not those that are serious or dangerous such as aggression, verbal abuse, stealing, and noncompliance. But if you're always blowing up, you are less likely to get compliance on the important issues, and you're reinforcing the minor ones with your attention.

In order to appropriately ignore a behavior that you expect will go away or diminish, you must make sure that you totally disregard it. Understand that it might get worse (or at least more frequent) before it gets better. Do not give in and start punishing it because you become frustrated. This approach will take practice and a consistency of its own.

NEGATIVE CONSEQUENCES

More serious and dangerous behaviors, especially those that represent noncompliance and rule violations, need to be linked to consistent and firm consequences. After you've received some training and support, you can use time-outs and the removing of rewards and privileges quite effectively with even a very difficult-to-raise ADHD youngster.

Spanking, however, should not be considered an option. Even if you feel pushed to the limit by your child's misbehavior, noncompliance, or aggression, never spank your child. Corporal punishment is an unacceptable option for disciplining ADHD children for several reasons.

First, ADHD children are often very physical, and spanking only encourages aggressive behavior. When your ADHD child sees you dealing with your frustration through spanking or hitting, he learns that this is the way to solve problems. In addition, he learns that it's all right for a big person to hit a smaller person to get what he wants.

Second, children with ADHD already suffer from low self-esteem. Hitting her could lead her to feel even more worthless. Your efforts in discipline and training should be to build your child's sense of worth.

Third, it may be difficult for some parents to draw the line between punishment and abuse. You may think you know how much spanking is excessive, but your child may not. When you spank in anger, you run the risk of inadvertently causing serious physical or emotional injury.

The bottom line is that spanking does not work. Most studies show that the consistency of punishment is more important than the intensity or type of punishment.[9] Other studies show that spanking and physical punishment lead to more aggression and hostility in children and often have psychological effects—such as depression and suicidal or abusive tendencies—that last into adolescence and adulthood.[10]

Many children need a combination of discipline methods in order to learn to keep their impulsivity and aggression under control. You can help your child learn self-control through your patience and calmness, providing structure, and using a combination of effective discipline methods. While ADHD children often need negative consequences to give them feedback about their noncompliant behavior, they also need the skills they can learn through such positive techniques as praise, attention, and rewards.

Goal 4: Take Care of Yourself

Using appropriate discipline and providing structure for your ADHD child can give you greater control over your family life. But constant efforts to handle a difficult and challenging child can wear you down unless you keep your own well-being in mind. Here are some strategies for easing your personal stress.

BUILD YOURSELF UP

If you're like most people, when you've been experiencing prolonged stress, you are less likely to take care of yourself. That generally translates into less concern about what you eat, with a consequent increase in weight. When you put on a few pounds, you tend to feel more sluggish, you exercise less, and you begin to feel more depressed. People who are depressed tend to exercise less, drink more alcohol, take more drugs, and smoke.[11] As a result, you suffer physically.

If this downward spiral sounds familiar, you have begun to target what you need to do to stop the self-defeating cycle and make positive changes.

Changing your attitude is the next step. Think of parenting an ADHD child in this way: You have an important, critical job facing you. You are going to deal with a challenging child on a daily basis for several years. You've accepted this challenge, and you're going to succeed at it. To do so, though, you must prepare.

You wouldn't think of running in a marathon, playing hockey in the NHL, or trying out for an Olympic swimming event without months of rigorous training, right? Why would you think that you can parent a very active, impulsive child without full preparation? When you look at it this way, you can see that your mental attitude is essential in training for the job ahead of you.

To begin your training, here's a list of things you must do:

• Make sure you are eating a healthy, balanced diet.

• Cut down or stop the use of alcohol, tobacco, or other substances that could interfere with your health or functioning.

• Exercise at least three times a week for thirty minutes.

• Learn some relaxation techniques. To put yourself in a relaxed, quiet mood, try listening to soothing classical music, or focus your imagination on a favorite vacation spot or a cherished childhood memory. Relaxation methods that have proven value include deep breathing, deep muscle relaxation, and Transcendental Meditation. Look for books and audio or videocassettes that teach one of these methods.

Keep encouraging yourself. Use positive self-talk or affirmations to keep yourself going and to ward off negative thoughts. In a distressing time, for instance, reaffirming to yourself that "I can get through this day" can be useful. Or, "I am a capable parent doing the best job I can" might be helpful in a public place when your child is misbehaving. Having a mantra of sorts to get you through the worst times can be especially useful. Some parents of ADHD children have said over and over again to themselves: "This too shall pass." Whatever you say to yourself, make sure it is positive, reassuring, and perhaps inspiring.

Be sure to develop other interests besides parenting your child. Your most important job may be that of a parent, but that can't be your whole life. Put some romance in your life, go on vacation, develop a hobby or part-time employment, and keep up with friends so you have someone to call when you need to talk to an adult.

It is very helpful to have an evacuation plan ready. Be prepared to get away from your ADHD child when the stress is intolerable. Work out arrangements with a relative, neighbor, or friend so that you can trade services. Taking a break from your child for only an hour or two can be useful in recharging your worn-out batteries.

AVOID ISOLATION

You need a social support network: a shoulder to cry on and someone to talk to at the moment when stress is greatest. Maybe you have a friend or relative who is willing to listen to you when you need to talk about your particularly trying day with your child. There are support groups and even chat lines on the Internet for parents of ADHD children.[12] Psychotherapy (as discussed in Chapter 10), can help too because it offers parents a safe environment where they can express and learn to cope with some of their most unpleasant feelings. No matter how much chaos, tension, and turmoil your child brings into your home, you don't have to suffer alone.

CHAPTER TWELVE

Educational Interventions

*I*f your child has ADHD, chances are your school is the place where the problems are the most evident.[1] In order to best identify the particular problems your child experiences and to develop a plan to handle them, you need to have a good working relationship with your child's teachers. Try to think of your child's teachers as your partners in his care, with each of you having special responsibilities.

Your Responsibility as a Parent

The plain fact is that you will have to be more involved in your ADHD child's education than a parent of a non-ADHD child might be. Many times parents—

whether of ADHD or non-ADHD children—don't realize the critical role they play in their children's academic achievement. Several studies have shown that parental participation is a more important factor in children's school progress than such things as the parents' level of education, their occupations, or the family's social or economic standing in the community.[2] T. M. Black perhaps said it best (although he wasn't referring specifically to parents of ADHD children) when he said, "We must guard against relinquishing basic responsibility for childrearing to society. . . . Being a parent . . . is a responsibility which can be shared with others—schools, day care centers—but should never be abandoned to them."[3]

As a parent, the first thing you need to do is to make sure the school is aware that your child has ADHD. You should:

• Provide the school with appropriate documentation, test reports, and medical information about your child.

• Arrange a meeting, in person if possible but at least on the phone, between the teacher and the physician.

• Provide the school with an appropriate amount of medication, and work out the details about how it will be administered.

• Let the teacher know when there are events in your child's life that will affect school performance.

- Attend school meetings.

- Design an appropriate study area at home.

- Set a consistent time for homework and study.

- Help with homework when needed.

- Praise your child's school efforts.

The School's Responsibilities

Wouldn't a great burden be lifted off your shoulders if you knew that your ADHD child was receiving special, individualized attention from a teacher? Wouldn't you sleep better at night if she had access to special computer games for reading comprehension and a partner to help her focus?

Most parents—even those who don't have a child with ADHD—would be delighted to have access to such classroom perks. The truth is, they're not necessarily such luxuries. Many school districts are taking a proactive approach to ADHD and are providing comprehensive training and support materials to teachers and support staff like nurses, social workers, and psychologists.

Teachers are recognizing the value of such training. "I want to deal with it, to face it," says "Becky Woodley," a grade-school teacher in a Detroit suburban school district where administrators have aggressively pursued ADHD training for teachers. "I welcome suggestions from parents about how to deal with their ADHD child." In the long run, Becky says, it's worth it to spend extra time addressing the needs of the children in her class.

"The nightmare is when there's a child with ADHD in your class and the parents just don't want to deal with it," adds Becky, "or they deny there's a problem. The whole class suffers then because of one student."

In classrooms around the country, ADHD students are benefiting from such practices as:

• *Lowered noise levels:* This simple adjustment can be a godsend to the ADHD student trying to focus on an assignment or a lesson.

• *Visualization techniques:* Many teachers are helping ADHD students absorb information by teaching them to close their eyes, relax, and visualize what is being read aloud.

• *Movement activities:* Jumping rope during a spelling lesson might sound strange, but for the ADHD child who quickly wearies of sitting at a desk, it's a stimulating way to learn.

These are just three of the teaching devices described in "101 Ways to Help Children with ADD Learn," a publication of the U.S. Department of Education.[4] The booklet is only one of many resources readily available to educators and parents. Many teachers will already be familiar with it and the many other teaching aids and resources for working with ADHD children. You may not be lucky enough to find a teacher with a lot of experience, or even much ADHD training, but chances are you'll find one who is open to suggestions and ideas.

"Mary Sanders" asked for a school meeting after her son "Mark," age ten, was diagnosed with ADHD. It took persistence, but finally Mary was able to coordinate a meeting at his elementary school with the principal, four teachers who had Mark in different classes, the school social worker, the school psychologist, and the psychologist from a mental health clinic where the ADHD assessment was carried out.

Mary came to the meeting with a copy of Mark's ADHD assessment, which included recommendations, a notebook in which she had written questions, and a determination that this meeting would not end until they had drawn up a workable plan for Mark.

To Mary's relief, Mark's teacher was familiar with ADHD and seemed committed to helping him in whatever way she could. His teacher also encouraged Mary to call her at home, or stop by the school anytime she had a concern or a question. She also agreed to make sure that Mark took all his graded assignments home so that his parents could evaluate his progress.

Mary asked the teacher if she would mind moving Mark to the front of the classroom, where he would have a clear view of the chalkboard and where distractions from other students would be kept to a minimum. The teacher was happy to do so.

Not all teachers are willing to agree to arrangements suggested by parents and school staff. Some teachers are either not flexible or unwilling to accommodate one or two ADHD students in the classroom. If this is the case with your child's school, then, like Mary, you have to become an advocate for your child to make sure his needs are being met.[5] As an advocate, you will have to be involved in monitoring your child's schoolwork, the completion of assignments, and his relationship with the teacher, and be ready to make suggestions to the teacher when you see a problem.

Sometimes, despite your best efforts, you will encounter an unresponsive or uncooperative teacher. Assuming that you have already solicited a partnership with the teacher, the next step will be to talk to the principal. You could request a change of teachers or ask that the principal act as a mediator between you and the teacher. If this step fails, the director of either elementary or secondary education (depending on the grade level of your child) is the next person to contact. A written request for assistance to an administrator at this level is often successful.

The Teacher's Responsibilities

The teacher's responsibilities are to:

• Understand and accept the child's disorder.

• Design a classroom environment in which the child can learn.

• Provide instruction that is interactive and enjoyable.

• Select classroom materials that are of high interest to children.

• Make classroom expectations, rules, consequences, and rewards very clear.

• Develop a behavior management system that is helpful to the ADHD child.

• Administer tests that allow the ADHD child to demonstrate his understanding of the material.

• Praise the child's efforts.

• Avoid statements and actions that bring attention to any child's disorder and disabilities.

WORKING WITH THE TEACHER TO ADDRESS EDUCATIONAL PROBLEMS

One immediate way that the teacher can help your child is to seat her up front. That is, the teacher can provide "proximity management," using the closeness of her presence or even touch to help keep your child's attention focused. Seating the child at the front of the classroom will also reduce her visual distractions, as most other students will not be in her line of vision. It will allow her to have direct eye contact with the teacher, who will be able to give visual or verbal cues to help her stay with tasks.

Teachers can also help an ADHD child by creating a distraction-free environment, an area of the classroom that is more isolated and uncluttered, where he can go on his own to work. Partitions, shields, and study carrels around desks help to cut down on the distractions in the typical classroom.

You might also provide the teacher with tokens or small incentives that she can use as tangible reinforcements for your child. The offer of a reward—even merit points that add up to some more immediate acknowledgment—can help children learn to stay with a task.[6] As the child stays with a task or activity, his focus on it is strengthened. The reward can be phased out eventually as attentiveness improves, especially if the teacher replaces it with plenty of verbal praise.

You and the teacher should work together to create a plan to help your child complete assignments on time and correctly. You might work out a home-school contract together, spelling out the expectations you and the teacher have for your child. The contract can specify not only when and how your child will do assignments, but also what reinforcements will be given as a reward for successful improvement.

For Mark Sanders, the home-school contract stated that he would do his schoolwork between four and five P.M. As a reward for completing this work, he would be allowed to play outside with friends until six-thirty, at which time he was to come in for dinner.

Some teachers and parents have found that a major part of ADHD children's difficulty with homework relates to poor organization skills.[7] Getting your child organized—by using color-coordinated class notebooks, assignment and homework folders, daily assignment sheets, and personal daily reminders—can make a difference. It will also help if you set up a regular homework and study time, providing a quiet, clutter-free area for study. You can monitor the completion of assignments, offer constructive feedback, and double-check the accuracy of all completed work.

Frequent parental monitoring, allowing short breaks from the study routine, and giving plenty of praise and attention can be most helpful in making sure your ADHD student completes her assignments and that they're ready to hand in the next day.

WORKING WITH THE TEACHER TO
ADDRESS BEHAVIORAL PROBLEMS

Your ADHD child is almost certain to have a short attention span and a high level of distractibility. In addition, she may well be hyperactive and impulsive. The consequences of these symptoms could be disruptive behavior that gets her into trouble at school.

"Tim Larson," a seven-year-old ADHD student, couldn't sit still in class. He seemed to bounce around the classroom and was constantly in the wrong place at the wrong time. If the other children were sitting in a circle to listen to the teacher read a story, Tim was standing by the window staring at the playground. If the other children were standing in line to go outdoors, Tim was in the art supply corner of the room twirling a pair of scissors on his fingers. This kind of behavior exasperated his teacher, who always had to be on the alert for where Tim was and what he was doing.

"Tracy Samuels," a nine-year-old ADHD child, behaved much as Tim did, but she was disruptive in more serious ways. When the teacher asked a question, instead of raising her hand to be called on, Tracy blurted out an answer. When children lined up, Tracy would push and shove other children out of her way. When another child annoyed or angered her, Tracy often responded with obscene language, pinching, poking with pencils, spitting, or hitting. Since these behaviors could not be tolerated, especially when the parents of other children complained to the principal, Tracy was frequently sent home.

Behavior problems such as those exhibited by Tim and Tracy are common among ADHD students and all involve difficulties with self-control. Because these difficulties occur at school, it is hard for parents to have a direct influence on them. By developing a partnership with your child's teacher, you can support each other's efforts to control the child's disruptive behavior, making sure that the same principles are applied at home and at school.

These principles include:

Positive feedback

All children, especially ADHD children, need positive encouragement and verbal praise. To teach a disruptive child better self-control, you should offer daily doses of praise, positive attention, compliments, and encouragement for desirable behaviors.

Clear and reasonable rules

Both at home and in the classroom, adults need to give children with impulse control problems clear, consistent, and reasonable expectations and rules. There should be no doubt in an ADHD child's mind as to what the rule is and whether that rule is in effect on any particular day.

Constructive negative feedback

Serious negative behaviors—whether at home or in the classroom—cannot be ignored. Both parents and teachers need to avoid addressing those behaviors in destructive and damaging ways, such as by yelling, nagging, sarcasm, or putdowns. Instead, try using nonverbal cues, signs, colored stickers, and the removal of points to give immediate and more constructive feedback about unacceptable behavior.

Consistent and firm consequences

The consequences of noncompliance, aggression, or other serious or dangerous misbehavior must be clear to your child. While constant punishment may eventually increase negative behavior, firm consequences such as time-outs and loss of privileges, consistently applied, can show the child which misbehaviors will not be tolerated and help him begin to earn positive feedback.[8]

Social skills development

Because ADHD seriously compromises self-control, your child may have problems with anger, aggression, empathy, and conflict resolution. One way your child can learn self-control is for the important adults in her life—you and her teacher—to teach her the social skills she needs. When a teacher shows her students by example how to control anger, how to act in an assertive rather than aggressive manner, and how to solve problems and conflicts calmly, she is teaching valuable lessons in social skills.

Written reports

Many teachers take it upon themselves to communicate with parents in writing on a weekly or bimonthly basis. Often these reports are sent home with the student, to be signed or initialed by the parents and returned. These reports, when they address such matters as performance and conduct, can help both parent and teacher monitor the child's progress and give positive reinforcement for good behavior. If your child's teacher isn't using this "Friday folder" routine, perhaps you could discuss the possibility.

Behavior modification

A behavior modification approach to helping an ADHD child involves giving rewards for acceptable behavior and withdrawing rewards for unacceptable behavior. Such an approach works best when the rewards for desirable behavior are immediate, when the reward is highly desired by the child, and when there are visual indications of success or failure. When a behavioral approach is used at home and at school, the chances of long-term success are enhanced.

RITALIN AND THE SCHOOL

Another important matter you and your child's teacher will have to work out is the administration of medication at school. Most Ritalin is prescribed in the short-acting form, which means, almost certainly, that secondary doses have to be dispensed at some point during the school day. Once upon a time the school nurse made sure school children received their medication, but budget cuts in most districts have all but eliminated this job or reduced nurses to part-time status. These days medical matters are, more often than not, tended to by secretaries and teachers. In many schools children are told to stop by the office during lunchtime for their "afternoon dose" of Ritalin.

Matt Lee, 12, has been taking Ritalin since first grade, and stopping by the office to see the secretary has long been merely a matter of routine.

"It's never worried us," says his mother, Jan. "I always make sure the medicine is taken to school in the prescription bottle with Matt's name on it. I know the secretary knows Matt, and she's very responsible."

Other parents may, understandably, feel less confident. They worry that secretaries will make mistakes if they're passing out pills to long lines of students, and they worry that their children won't remember to get their medication. If you're one of these parents, you should certainly try to develop a different plan. If a school nurse isn't available, perhaps the teacher would be willing to monitor the procedure. Randy Phillips, for example, has his second dose delivered to his kindergarten room. His mother, Susan, is happy about the arrangement because the burden isn't on her six-year-old to make sure he gets his medication.

If your child will be taking Ritalin or other medication at school, you should:

• Make a personal visit to the school and meet with the teacher, the principal, and anyone else who will be involved in making sure your child receives her medication.

• Find out what the backup plan is if the teacher or secretary is absent. Who will be dispensing medication on these days?

• Never allow your child to take his pill on his own, no matter how old or responsible he is. If your child is caught with Ritalin, a controlled substance, she could be subject to some harsh disciplinary action.

Special Classes

Some ADHD children function well in a regular classroom. It has been estimated that 65 percent of children with the disorder will remain in mainstream classes and will, with assistance and accommodation, succeed.[9]

Other ADHD children have serious enough learning problems—in spelling, reading, math, or handwriting—that they need the extra help of special education classes. Children cannot be considered for special education classes without a rigorous series of steps and tests, which will be governed by the laws in your state, as well as approval from you. If your child does qualify for special education services, an individual education plan (IEP), usually requested by the teacher, will be developed by an IEP team (usually consisting of the teacher, the school psychologist, education specialists, and the parents). It will spell out in writing specifically what your child's problems are, what the goals are, and what services the school will offer to meet the goals. In short, an IEP is a program or plan for educating your child based on his individual needs.

Implementing an IEP requires your written consent. If you have second thoughts or feel that you have been pressured into signing something you don't agree with, you will have a specified amount of time to change your mind.

It may also be reassuring to know that each year the IEP team will meet again to review progress and

alter the plan if it is not succeeding or meeting your
child's needs.

Alternative Educational Plans

Despite your best efforts and the most cooperative relationship between you and the teacher, it's possible
that your child will not fit in at a public school, even in
a special education program.

A private school may be an alternative, if you have
the financial resources. Many schools throughout the
country now offer special curricula for ADHD children
and young adults, even up to the college level.

Some parents have found home schooling to be a
viable alternative. A word of caution here: Home-
schooling is not something to be undertaken lightly. It
requires an enormous effort from you and your child,
as well as a commitment to discipline that few are
willing to make. If you have little patience for working with your child or if you have serious discipline
problems with her, you should think long and hard
about undertaking this task. Then too, as Mike Merz, a
school psychologist in Oakland County, Michigan, re-
minds parents, ADHD is a lifelong disorder, and your
child is going to have to figure out a way to get along
in the world. Part of the school's role, he says, "is to
prepare the child to fit in to society and to learn to accommodate others."[10]

But for some people, it is a viable option. Elaine

and "John Dunbar" home-school four of their five children, four of whom have varying degrees of ADHD.

"They were miserable in the public school," says Elaine. "They concentrate so much better at home because my environment is not distracting to them."

Elaine admits it is a task but not one without rewards. "I celebrate a lot of victories with them I'd miss otherwise," she says. "In fact, if they were still in school, they'd probably miss them, too."

It doesn't cost anything to take an active role in your child's education, and your involvement will be a major factor in his eventual educational success. By establishing a supportive and positive partnership with your child's school, you increase his chances for academic success.

CHAPTER THIRTEEN

The Big Picture: Adults with ADHD

*F*or years ADHD was considered to be a problem specific to children and adolescents.[1] Many experts mistakenly believed it was entirely behavioral, and that time and maturity would eventually offer blessed relief.

By the 1980s, however, the vast amount of research that had accumulated on ADHD made it clear that the disorder is physiological—that somewhere in the brain of the ADHD individual, the neurotransmitters are failing to do their jobs. This evidence posed a problem: Why would the imbalance suddenly reverse itself during adulthood?

The answer is that it doesn't. ADHD is one of the fastest-growing diagnoses of adults in the United States.[2] In 1993 the national support group CHADD officially changed its name from Children with Attention Deficit Disorders to Children and Adults with Attention Deficit Disorders. In the past five years, adult ADHD support groups have sprouted across the country.

Recognizing ADHD in Adults

If you are aware that you have ADHD, you either began treatment for it as a child—perhaps in the 1970s and 1980s—or you have been assessed recently and diagnosed. Many times adults become aware of the disorder in themselves when it is discovered in one of their children.

Susan Phillips says she and her husband, Sean, were so anxious about the results of their son's ADHD assessment that they asked for a special meeting with the child psychiatrist. The first thing the doctor did was hand them a checklist.

"I started filling it out for Randy," Susan says, "and I began thinking, 'This is my husband' and 'Oh my God, this is me.'"

Many appointments and many months later, Susan's suspicions were confirmed. All three Phillipses were diagnosed with ADHD.

Ritalin itself has generated a great deal of press in the past fifteen years, and this publicity has led many adults to learn more about ADHD and to evaluate themselves for symptoms. "Lawrence Hilliard" fought the symptoms of ADHD for forty years before he spot-

ted the headline "Ritalin Successes ADD Up" in a
daily newspaper.

"It was the first time I ever read about attention
deficit disorder," he recalls, and it led him to seek help.

If you grew up knowing you had ADHD—and
dealing with it—you've got an obvious advantage.
For the adults who don't discover it until later in
life, years of failure and frustration have often taken
their toll.

Frank Lee was diagnosed with ADHD when he
was in his forties. A few months later he was diagnosed
with depression. The diagnoses were not surprising
after years of feeling inadequate, Frank says. "I still
can't get over the feeling that I wasted so much of
my life."

How ADHD Feels

ADHD appears somewhat different in adults than
in children. For one thing, hyperactivity—one of the
most common symptoms of ADHD in children—is
rarely a problem for adults because it's the easiest
symptom to learn to live with.[3] By the time you ma-
ture, you've probably figured out how to channel your
hyperactivity into exercise or sports, or you might have
a job that requires a lot of physical energy. For adults
who have learned to channel it, hyperactivity can actually be an asset.

Other symptoms, such as inattention, poor concentration, and impulsivity are a different story. For the

adult who can't finish a project, or even get organized enough to start one, life can be one chronic frustration. ADHD adults are impatient and sometimes hot tempered. "I always thought I was probably just crazy," says Susan Phillips, who was diagnosed at 35. "It wasn't just at school and at work. I couldn't even pay attention long enough to clean my house," she says. "I spent so many years being called a scatterbrain that I just resigned myself to that role."

Professionally you may be so disorganized that you fail at assignments or projects. You may find it difficult, or even impossible, to sit at your desk long enough to complete jobs.

Frank Lee landed a lot of sales-type jobs in his thirty-five years in the workforce. He lost a lot of them, too. "I could sell, but I couldn't pay attention long enough to complete a form," he says.

Impulsivity generally doesn't wear too well in the workplace, either. Hot tempers and emotional outbursts are simply not acceptable professional decorum. Sometimes no amount of apologizing can undo the damage caused by inappropriate or inconsiderate remarks.

Impulsive adults also are renowned for making snap decisions. "I'd quit a job in the blink of an eye," says Frank. "I never stopped to consider the consequences, like how my family was going to survive without my income."

These behaviors can thwart friendships and strain or destroy marriages. Not remembering to pick up the cleaning or empty the trash doesn't seem like a crime.

But when such offenses occur again and again, they can wreak havoc on even the healthiest relationship.

Julie Ogg sometimes got the feeling her husband, Steve, just didn't care. "Steve's problems were so frustrating," she says. "He wouldn't be aware things needed to be done. He'd just forget."

When Steve would make a phone call and then forget who he'd called before they answered, it was funny at first. Then it got irritating.

When the frustration levels got so bad that their relationship began to show some wear and tear, the Oggs took themselves to a marriage counselor. The counselor got right to the point. She suggested that Steve be assessed for ADHD. And when the diagnosis came, it was a blessing. It gave Julie and Steve something to work on, something tangible to fix.

It may not be clear—even to you—how ADHD is affecting you. Children are always in classrooms with teachers as skilled observers, but for adults there are few such controlled environments where the deficits caused by ADHD can be objectively measured.

Adult Assessment

The same thoroughgoing team approach that is used to diagnose ADHD in children—excluding the teacher observation, of course—is essential for diagnosing ADHD in adults. One reason is that far more adults with ADHD suffer from the various related disorders, such as depression and anxiety, than children do.[4]

When Sean Phillips was diagnosed with ADHD, he had no idea he was also carrying around the additional baggage of an anxiety disorder. "First I was diagnosed with ADHD," he says, "and Ritalin made a world of difference. But there was still something wrong."

He began regular psychotherapy, and eventually his doctor prescribed Prozac in addition to Ritalin.

"I couldn't believe it," Sean says. "For the first time in my life, this ache in my gut was gone."

Treatment

As Sean's experience shows, a multimodal treatment program, combining psychotherapy with medication, is as critical for adults as it is for children. Though Ritalin often plays a primary role in adult therapy, it appears to be less effective for them than it is for children and adolescents.[5] The changes Ritalin produces may seem less dramatic in adults because they are overshadowed by other problems or because adults may have learned, over time, how to manage some of their ADHD symptoms.

Adults also seem to have more problems dealing with the drug's side effects and stigma.[6] When his doctor suggested that he needed to take Ritalin, Steve Ogg recalls, "I was embarrassed and humiliated."

"Steve had low self-esteem," says his wife, Julie. "He was very defensive about all this."

Steve eventually did take Ritalin, though, and started behavior modification therapy. Since then, his life has turned around. He went to school, completed his degree, and received an impressive promotion at work. The Oggs also started their own business.

Steve gives Ritalin a lot of credit for his success, but he still has trouble coping with its side effects. He says it makes him jittery when he first takes it, then grouchy when it wears off.

Susan Phillips tolerated Ritalin well from the start. But she didn't realize just how much it was affecting her until she went on vacation—and forgot her pills. "For the whole week, I felt completely out of control," she says. "It ruined the whole trip."

Ritalin helps most adults—at least 60 percent—control the symptoms of ADHD. But if you're an adult with ADHD, the major focus of treatment should be on rebuilding your self-esteem and confidence and eliminating some of the roadblocks that have interfered with your professional, social, and intimate relationships. Psychotherapy can offer help with these issues, but it's also critically important to enlist the people in your life in your treatment plan. Children, after all, have mothers and fathers and teachers to coach them every day. You need a coach, too—someone who can offer you guidance and encouragement on a regular basis and who can help you translate positive thoughts and ideas into action. Your coach could be your therapist, your spouse, a friend, or a support group colleague who is also dealing with the disorder. If you have a child who is grown, perhaps he could fill this critical coaching role.

Having a coach doesn't relieve you of the responsibilities of dealing with your ADHD. No one can do the work for you. Your coach, however, could help you:

• Plan and set goals.

• Work on concentration and time management skills.

• Develop a network of supportive people.

• Practice social skills.

Susan and Sean Phillips coach each other. He calls her several times during the day for a mutual support session. They don't just keep a calendar, they discuss their plans on a weekly basis. They attend CHADD meetings together and talk to other parents and adults about ADHD. "The Ritalin helps us each manage our minute-to-minute problems," Susan says, "but coaching each other helps us manage our whole lives."

The Long-Term Impact of ADHD on Adults

The outlook for adults with ADHD can be excellent, assuming that they are properly diagnosed and treated.

Frank Lee resents the time he lost to ADHD, but finally, thanks to psychotherapy and medication, he is able to focus more on the future than on the past. He's now managed to stay in one job long enough to build up seniority and even a pension.

Susan Phillips has almost completed the coursework necessary to receive her master's degree. And, she is proud to claim, she has managed to keep her house clean while studying.

Steve Ogg has continued behavior modification, which he loves, and Ritalin, which he doesn't.

"You have to figure out where you are on a continuum when you have ADHD," he says. "If you keep running into roadblocks, you need some help."

He hopes to move along the continuum to the point where he no longer needs medication. In the meantime he's happy with where he's at. "I'm controlling my ADHD," Steve says. "It's not controlling me."

NOTES

Chapter One: What Is Ritalin?

1. S. E. Shaywitz and B. A. Shaywitz, "Attention Deficit Disorder: Diagnosis and Role of Ritalin in Management," *Ritalin: Theory and Patient Management* (New York: Mary Ann Liebert, 1992), p. 45.

2. R. A. Barkley, "Attention Deficit Hyperactivity Disorder," *Psychiatric Annals.* vol. 21, no. 12 (1991), pp. 725–33.

3. J. D. Lawrence, D. B. Lawrence, and D. S. Caron, "Optimizing ADHD Therapy with Sustained-Release Methylphenidate," *American Family Physician,* vol. 55, no. 5 (1997), pp. 1705–09 (at 1705).

4. "Methylphenidate," DEA press release (Washington, D.C.: September 13, 1995), p. 1.

5. David Treadwell, "Parents Challenge Hyperactivity Drug for Children," *Los Angeles Times;* in *Detroit News*, December 29, 1987.

6. G. J. DuPaul and R. A. Barkley, "Medication Therapy," *Attention Deficit Hyperactivity Disorder: A Handbook for Diagnosis and Treatment* (New York: Guilford Press, 1991), p. 589. The authors state that all stimulant medications can produce "temporary symptoms of psychosis at very high doses, or even at smaller doses in very young children (below the ages of 3 or 4 years of age)." But they consider a psychotic reaction to be a highly unique side effect.

7. N. D. Volkow, et al., "Is Methylphenidate Like Cocaine? Studies on their Pharmacokinetics and Distribution in the Human Brain," *Archives of General Psychiatry,* vol. 52 (1995), pp. 456–63. The authors conclude that the pharmacokinetics (bodily absorption, distribution, metabolism, and excretion) of methylphenidate and cocaine differ markedly. Essentially, the "high" experienced when methylphenidate is taken intranasally decreases rapidly compared with cocaine.

8. Barkley, "Attention Deficit," quoted in a Scripps-Howard news service story by John Lang, June 1997.

9. "Attention Deficit Disorder—Part II," *Harvard Mental Health Letter,* vol. 11, no. 11 (May 1995), p. 1.

10. *Physicians' Desk Reference* (Montvale, NJ: Medical Economics Company, 1997); hereinafter *PDR.*

11. "Methylphenidate," DEA press release (September 1995), p. 1.

12. D. J. Safer, J. M. Zito, and E. M. Fine, "Increased Methylphenidate Usage for Attention Deficit Disorder in the 1990s," *Pediatrics,* vol. 98 (1986), pp. 1084–88. The se-

nior author of this study, Safer, has been doing prevalence studies for at least fifteen years; he and his coauthors in this article report that between 1990 and 1995 there has been a 2.5-fold increase in the prevalence of methylphenidate treatment of youths with ADHD. This data tends to correct exaggerated media claims of a sixfold expansion of methylphenidate treatment. The authors' conclusion is that 2.8 percent (or 1.5 million) of American youth ages 5 to 18 were receiving this treatment in 1995.

13. J. M. Halperin, J. H. Newcorn, and V. Sharma, "Ritalin: Diagnostic Comorbidity and Attentional Measures," *Ritalin: Theory and Patient Management* (New York: Mary Ann Liebert, 1992), p. 20.

14. *PDR.*

15. Shaywitz and Shaywitz, "Attention Deficit Disorder."

16. Dr. Ruth Robin, at a CHADD meeting, Oxford, Michigan, November 13, 1995.

17. V. S. Cowart, "The Ritalin Controversy: What's Made this Drug's Opponents Hyperactive?" *Journal of the American Medical Association,* vol. 259, no. 17 (May 6, 1988), pp. 2521–23. "Howard McClain, chief of drug control in the Office of Diversion Control of the Drug Enforcement Agency, said that the big increase [in manufacture of Ritalin] between 1985 and 1986 [an increase of 682 kilos, as compared to increases of 200 kilos or less in previous years], was due more to the market entry of a second generic manufacturer than to a sudden surge in the amount of the drug sold, although that also has increased over the five-year period. A Ciba-Geigy Corporation [the company that manufactured Ritalin at that time] spokesman said that, for several years before the increase in the amount manufactured,

the company was unable to fill all its orders for methylphenidate with the amount available."

18. Daniel J. Safer, M.D., "Medication Usage Trends for ADD," *Attention*, vol. 2, no. 2 (Fall 1995), pp. 11–15.

19. C. Y. Alston and D. M. Romney, "A Comparison of Medicated and Nonmedicated Attention Deficit Disordered Hyperactive Boys," *Acta Paedopsychiatrica: International Journal of Child and Adolescent Psychiatry*, vol. 55, no. 2 (1992), pp. 65–70.

20. R. A. Barkley, "The Effects of Methylphenidate on the Interactions of Pre-school ADHD Children with their Mothers," *Journal of the American Academy of Child and Adolescent Psychiatry*, vol. 27, no. 3 (1988), pp. 336–41.

21. V. I. Douglas, et al., "Short-Term Effects of Methylphenidate on the Cognitive Learning and Academic Performance of Children with Attention Deficit Disorder in the Laboratory and the Classroom," *Journal of Child Psychology and Psychiatry and Allied Disciplines*, vol. 27, no. 2 (1986), pp. 191–211.

22. M. Lechner, "Attention Deficit Hyperactivity Disorder," *Clinical Update*, Hurley Medical Center (Flint, Michigan), vol. 2, no. 4 (n.d.), p. 1.

23. Andrew R. Adesman, M.D., and Esther H. Wender, M.D., "Improving the Outcome for Children with ADHD," *Contemporary Pediatrics* (March 1991), pp. 122–39.

24. E. Susman, "What Do You Say to Ritalin?" *Edge* (Jan.–Feb., 1996), p. 1.

Chapter Two: What Is ADHD?

1. American Psychiatric Association, *Diagnostic and Statistical Manual of Mental Disorders* (Washington D.C.: American Psychiatric Association, 1994); hereinafter *DSM-IV*. This publication indicates that the estimated prevalence of ADHD in children is 3 to 5 percent. It also says that the prevalence among adolescents and adults is unknown because the data is "limited."

A review of the research indicates that the estimates range from 1 to 20 percent, depending on the rigor of the criteria used to define the disorder. See D. M. Ross and S. A. Ross, *Hyperactivity: Current Issues, Research, and Theory* (New York: John Wiley, 1982).

A study of more than 14,000 Canadian schoolchildren reported prevalance statistics of 21 percent for boys and 7 percent for girls. See R. L. Tries et al., "Incidence of Hyperactivity," *Journal of Pediatric Psychology,* vol. 4 (1979), pp. 179–88.

Based on their own research, carried out and reported in the professional literature since 1986, Shaywitz and Shaywitz estimate that 10 to 20 percent of the school-age population is affected by ADHD. See B. A. Shaywitz and S. E. Shaywitz, "Attention Deficit Disorder: Diagnosis and Role of Ritalin in Management," *Ritalin: Theory and Patient Management* (New York: Mary Ann Liebert, 1992).

2. R. A. Barkley, *Attention Deficit Hyperactivity Disorder: A Handbook for Diagnosis* (New York: Guilford Press, 1990).

3. In the 1940s Strauss and his associates began to label children with behavior disorders as "brain damaged." In the 1950s other investigators began using the concept of "brain dysfunction" rather than "brain damage." "Minimal brain

dysfunction" was the preferred term into the 1960s. In 1980 *DSM-III* included "attention deficit disorder" as a specific diagnostic category for the first time. A few years later, when *DSM-III-Revised* was published, the name was changed to "attention deficit hyperactivity disorder." See Shaywitz and Shaywitz, "Attention Deficit Disorder."

4. Shaywitz and Shaywitz, "Attention Deficit Disorder."

5. R. McGee, et al., "A Twelve-Year Follow-Up of Preschool Hyperactive Children," *Journal of the American Academy of Child and Adolescent Psychiatry,* vol. 30, no. 2 (1991), pp. 224–32. This twelve-year follow-up study found preschoolers identified as "pervasively hyperactive" to continue to show poorer cognitive skills, lower levels of reading ability, disruptive and inattentive behaviors at home and at school, and higher rates of *DSM-III* disorders during preadolescence and adolescence. By age 15, only 25 percent of this group were identified as having met "recovery" criteria.

A review of the literature indicated that by early adulthood ADHD appeared to remain present in at least 30 percent of the subjects. See N. Lie, "Follow-Ups of Children With Attention Deficit Hyperactivity Disorder: Review of the Literature," *Acta Psychiatrica Scandinavica,* vol. 368 (1992), pp. 1–40.

In another study the authors followed ADHD children from ages 6–12 until they were 18–25. "Nearly half of the hyperactive children in the two studies outgrew the disorder completely and became normal adults. Thirty-one percent still had all the main symptoms of ADHD at 18, and more than 60 percent had at least one of the disabling symptoms at 24." See Gabrielle Weiss and Lily Hechtman, "What Happens to Hyperactive Children When They Grow Up?" *Harvard Mental Health Letter* (October 1989).

6. *DSM-IV* estimates that the ratio of boys to girls having ADHD ranges from 4:1 to 9:1. The National Institute of Mental Health (NIMH) says the ratio is 3:1. See S. Neuwirth, *Attention Deficit Hyperactivity Disorder: Decade of the Brain,* NIMH publication no. 94-3572 (Washington, D.C.: U.S. Government Printing Office, 1994).

7. Dianne Hales and Dr. Robert E. Hales, "Finally I Know What's Wrong," *Parade* (January 7, 1996), pp. 9–11. Dr. Edward Hallowell is quoted in this story as saying, "The formal diagnosis is attention deficit hyperactivity disorder, but not all patients—women in particular—show symptoms of hyperactivity."

8. "Another theory was that refined sugar and food additives make children hyperactive and inattentive. . . . After studying the data, the scientists concluded that the restricted diet only seemed to help about 5 percent of children with ADHD, mostly either young children or children with food allergies. . . . ADHD is not usually caused by too much TV, food allergies, excess sugar, poor home life, poor schools." Neuwirth, "Attention Deficit."

Currently the hypothesis that sugar ingestion leads to excessive activity has little empirical support. In one study, thirty-one mothers who believed their sons (ages five to seven) were behaviorally affected by sugar were randomly assigned to a sugar-expectancy group or a control group. Mothers in the sugar-expectancy group were told that their children had received a large dose of sugar. In the control group, mothers were told that their children had received a drink flavored with NutraSweet and that NutraSweet does not affect children behaviorally. In fact, all the children in both groups had received drinks flavored with aspartame. Mothers in the sugar-expectancy group rated their sons as more hyperactive in subsequent play sessions. All the boys wore wrist and ankle actometers during the play, which showed that boys in the sugar-expectancy group were actually less active than boys in the control group. D. W. Hoover and R. Milich, "Effects of Sugar Ingestion Expectancies on Mother-Child Interactions," *Journal of Abnormal Child Psychology,* vol. 22 (1994), pp. 501–15.

Judith Rapoport, M.D., director of the Child Psychiatry Division of the National Institute of Mental Health, says, "Every well-controlled study has shown that there is no link between sugar and behavior. This is absolutely a dead issue." Quoted in *Baltimore Sun* (February 3, 1994).

9. In one study ADHD children did poorer than non-ADHD children on standard intelligence tests. S. V. Faraone et al., "Intellectual Performance and School Failure in Children with Attention Deficit Hyperactivity Disorder and in their Siblings." *Journal of Abnormal Psychology,* vol. 102, no. 4 (1993), pp. 616–23.

According to *DSM-IV,* however, "Intellectual development, as assessed by individual IQ tests, appears to be somewhat lower in children with this disorder."

10. *DSM-IV.*

11. Barkley, *Attention Deficit.* See also A. C. D'Antoni, "Mystery or Mastery: Teaching Goal-Directed Persistence," *ADHD Report,* vol. 3 (1995), pp. 7–8.

12. Patricia H. Latham's remarks are recorded in *Proceedings of the CH.A.D.D. 1994 Annual Conference, Attention Deficit Disorders: A Global Perspective* (Fairfax, VA: Caset Associated, 1995).

13. Barkley, *Attention Deficit.*

14. M. A. Carskadon, S. M. Pueschel, and R. P. Millman, "Sleep-Disordered Breathing and Behavior in Three Risk Groups: Preliminary Findings from Parental Reports," *Child's Nervous System,* vol. 9, no. 8 (1993), pp. 452–57.

15. E. Tirosh et al., "Effect of Methylphenidate on Sleep in Children with Attention Deficit Hyperactivity Disorder: An Activity Monitor Study," *American Journal of Diseases of Children,* vol. 147, no. 12 (1993), pp. 1313–15.

16. Barkley, *Attention Deficit.*

17. *DSM-IV.*

18. Russell Barkley states that the coexistence of ADHD with other behavioral and emotional disorders is "generally quite common with up to 44% having at least one other psychiatric disorder." Over 50 percent of ADHD children have significant problems in social relationships with other children. R. A. Barkley, "Attention Deficit Hyperactivity Disorder," *Psychiatric Annals,* vol. 21, no. 12 (1991), p. 730.

Chapter Three: The Causes of ADHD

1. T. J. Willis and I. Lovaas, "A Behavioral Approach to Treating Hyperactive Children: The Parent's Role," in J. B. Millichap, ed., *Learning Disabilities and Related Disorders* (Chicago: Yearbook Medical, 1977), pp. 119–40.

2. Benjamin Feingold, *Why Your Child Is Hyperactive* (New York: Random House, 1974). The Feingold diet, proposed in the book as a way of coping with hyperactive and ADHD children, involved the removal of artificial flavoring, coloring,

and synthetic preservatives from daily meals. Feingold contended that these additives resulted in hyperactive behavior in children.

James Windell interviewed Dr. Feingold in 1980 and asked him about the success rate of his diet. "In our experience, we run about 60 to 70 percent good responses in children who are disturbed (hyperactive)," Feingold said.

3. L. Smith, *Your Child's Behavior Chemistry* (New York: Random House, 1975).

4. C. K. Conners, "Sugars and Hyperactivity," *Sugars and Sweeteners* (Boca Raton: CRC Press, 1991).

5. The Feingold Associations of the United States (FAUS) continues to publish a newsletter for members called *Pure Facts*. For information contact FAUS, P.O. Box 6550, Alexandria, VA 22306.

6. In 1983 James Windell interviewed various proponents of diet *and* medication remedies for ADHD. He was told that there were "100-plus" Feingold Associations across the country. At that time association members estimated that more than 200,000 children and adults were following the diet. James Windell, "Hyperactivity Debate Running Strong," *Detroit Free Press,* November 17, 1983.

According to the 1997 *Encyclopedia of Associations*, the Feingold Associations of the United States claims thirty local groups. A spokesperson for FAUS says that numerous children and adults are following the diet but no exact figures, or even estimates, are available.

7. "Diet and Hyperkinesis—An Update," *Journal of the American Dietetic Association,* vol. 83, no. 2 (August 1986).

8. D. Behar et al., "Sugar Challenge Testing with Children Considered Behaviorally 'Sugar Reactive,' " *Nutrition Behavior,* vol. 1, no. 277 (1984).

9. D. W. Hoover, "Effects of Sugar Ingestion Expectancies on Mother-Child Interactions," *Journal of Abnormal Psychology,* vol. 22 (1994), pp. 501–15.

10. C. Keith Connors, *Feeding the Brain: How Foods Affect Children* (New York: Plenum, 1984) and "How Food Affects Behavior and Learning in Children," *CHADDER* (Spring/ Summer 1990), pp. 10–11.

11. S. Neuwirth, *Attention Deficit Hyperactivity Disorder: Decade of the Brain,* National Institute of Mental Health publication no. 94–3572 (Washington, D.C.; U.S. Government Printing Office, 1994).

In 1982 the National Institutes of Health held a major scientific conference to discuss the issue of refined sugar and food additives as a cause of children's hyperactivity and inattentiveness. After studying the data, the scientists concluded that a restricted diet seemed to help only about 5 percent of children with ADHD. Those children who were helped seemed mostly to be young children or children with food allergies.

Alan Zametkin, senior staff psychiatrist of the Clinical Brain Imaging Section at the National Institute of Mental Health, says, "However, dietary sugar has little impact on cerebral glucose metabolism. There is minimal support for a relationship, if any, that exists between diet and hyperactivity." A. Zametkin, "The Neurobiology of Attention-Deficit Hyperactivity Disorder," *CHADDER* (Spring/Summer 1991), pp. 10–11.

12. J. M. Daly, et al., "The Relationship Between Childhood Asthma and Attention Deficit Hyperactivity Disorder: A Review of the Literature," *Journal of Attention Disorders,* vol. 1, no. 1 (1996), pp. 31–40.

13. Ibid

14. These claims have been made at various times to the authors during patient interviews. They also appear in the literature distributed by CHADD. For specific information: Internet site: "Controversial Treatments for Children with Attention Deficit Disorder," www. Chadd.org

15. R. A. Barkley, *Attention Deficit Hyperactivity Disorder: A Handbook for Diagnosis and Treatment* (New York: Guilford Press, 1990).

16. Barkley (1990), D. M. Ross, and S. A. Ross, *Hyperactivity: Current Issues, Research, and Theory* (New York: Guilford Press, 1981); D. K. Routh, "Hyperactivity," in P. Magrab, ed., *Psychological Management of Pediatric Problems* (Baltimore: University Park Press, 1978), pp. 3–78; E. A. Taylor, ed., *The Overactive Child* (Philadelphia: J.P. Lippincott, 1986); and M. O'Dougherty, K. H. Neuchterlain, and B. Drew, "Hyperactive and Hypoxic Children: Signal Detection, Sustained Attention, and Behavior," *Journal of Abnormal Psychology,* vol. 93 (1984), pp. 178–91.

17. E. H. Cook, et al., "Association of Attention Deficit Disorder and the Dopamine Transporter Gene," *American Journal of Human Genetics,* vol. 56, no. 4 (1995), pp. 993–98.

18. Peter Gorner of *Chicago Tribune*, in *Detroit Free Press* (April 11, 1995).

19. S. Neuwirth, *Attention Deficit*. In one study children at risk for ADHD were determined to be the offspring of adults

who were diagnosed as having childhood onset of ADHD. Fifty-seven percent of the at-risk children met the criterion for ADHD, even though 75 percent of them had been treated for ADHD. J. Biederman "High Risk for Attention Deficit Hyperactivity Disorder Among Children of Parents with Childhood Onset of the Disorder: A Pilot Study," *American Journal of Psychiatry,* vol. 152, no. 3 (1995), pp. 431–35.

20. S. V. Faraone, J. Biederman, and S. Milberger, "An Exploratory Study of ADHD Among Second-Degree Relatives of ADHD Children," *Biological Psychiatry,* vol. 35 (1994), pp. 398–402; and J. Biederman, et al., "Family-Genetic and Psychosocial Risk Factors in *DSM-III* Attention Deficit Disorder," *Journal of the American Academy of Child and Adolescent Psychiatry,* vol. 29, no. 4 (1990), pp. 526–33.

21. F. Levy, et al., "Attention Deficit Hyperactivity Disorder: A Category or a Continuum? Genetic Analysis of a Large-Scale Twin Study," *Journal of the American Academy of Child and Adolescent Psychiatry,* vol. 36, no. 6 (1997), pp. 737–44.

22. S. V. Faraone, et al., "An Exploratory Study of ADHD."

23. K. G. Sieg, et al., "SPECT Brain Imaging Abnormalities in Attention Deficit Hyperactivity Disorder," *Clinical Nuclear Medicine,* vol. 20, no. 1 (1995), pp. 55–60; and C. L. Bowden, C. K. Deutsch, and J. M. Swanson, "Plasma Dopamine-Beta-Hydroxylase and Platelet Monoamine Oxidase in Attention Deficit Disorder and Conduct Disorder," *Journal of the American Academy of Child and Adolescent Psychiatry,* vol. 27 (1988), pp. 171–74.

24. A. Zametkin, "Neurobiology."

25. K. G. Sieg, et al., "SPECT Brain Imaging."

26. J. Rapoport, et al., "Subtle Brain Circuit Abnormalities Confirmed in ADHD," National Institute of Mental Health press release, July 15, 1996. Reported study appeared in *Archives of General Psychiatry* (July 1996).

27. D. E. Comings and B. G. Comings, "Tourette's Syndrome and Attention Deficit Disorder with Hyperactivity: Are They Genetically Related?" *Journal of the American Academy of Child Psychiatry,* vol. 23, no. 2 (1984), pp. 138–46.

28. E. R. Knell and D. E. Comings, "Tourette's Syndrome and Attention Deficit Hyperactivity Disorder: Evidence for a Genetic Relationship." *Journal of Clinical Psychiatry,* vol. 54, no. 9 (1993), pp. 331–37; W. S. Matthews, "Attention Deficits and Learning Disabilities in Children with Tourette's Syndrome," *Psychiatric Annals,* vol. 18, no. 7 (1993), pp. 414–16; and D. L. Pauls, J. F. Leckman, and D. J. Cohen, "Familial Relationship Between Giles de la Tourette's Syndrome, Attention Deficit Disorder, Learning Disabilities, Speech Disorders, and Stuttering." *Journal of the American Academy of Child and Adolescent Psychiatry,* vol. 32, no. 5 (1993), pp. 1044–50.

29. "Questions and Answers About Tourette's Syndrome," *Tourette's Syndrome Association,* on Internet (www.bixler.com/brainnet/tourette.htm) (1996).

30. Ibid

31. B. K. Caparulo, et al., "Computed Tomographic Brain Scanning in Children with Developmental Neuropsychiatric Disorders," *Annual Progress in Child Psychiatry and Child Development* (1982), pp. 550–68.

   B. S. Peterson, "Neuroimaging in Child and Adolescent Neuropsychiatric Disorders," *Journal of the American*

Academy of Child and Adolescent Psychiatry, vol. 34 (1995), pp. 1560–76.

32. One study found no serious evidence that Ritalin affects the severity of tic disorders, but it may slightly increase the frequency of motor tics while decreasing vocal tics. K. D. Gadow, et al., "Efficacy of Methylphenidate for Attention Deficit Hyperactivity Disorder in Children with Tic Disorder," *Archives of General Psychiatry,* vol. 52 (1995), pp. 444–55.

33. Ibid. The authors conclude that methylphenidate may be safely used in the majority of children with ADHD and tic disorders.

Chapter Four: The ADHD Assessment

1. Robert Resnick, Ph.D., was interviewed by James Windell on July 13, 1995, and in two follow-up interviews.

2. Randall Edwards, "Is Hyperactivity Label Applied Too Frequently?" *Monitor* (January 1995), pp. 44–45.

3. The authors of one study report that children diagnosed with ADHD had more depression and anxiety than a matched group of children. Their results underscore the need for future studies to carefully assess children diagnosed with ADHD for other psychiatric symptoms. See P. S. Jensen, et al., "Anxiety and Depressive Disorders in Attention Deficit Disorder with Hyperactivity: New Findings," *American Journal of Psychiatry,* vol. 150, no. 8 (1993), pp. 1203–09. See also J. Biederman, et al., "Psychiatric Comorbidity Among Juveniles with Major Depression: Fact or

Artifact?" *Journal of the American Academy of Child and Adolescent Psychiatry,* vol. 34 (1995), pp. 579–90.

4. R. A. Barkley, "Diagnosis and Assessment of Attention Deficit Hyperactivity Disorder," *Comprehensive Mental Health Care,* vol. 1, no. 1 (1991), pp. 27–43; G. L. Martin, "Assessment Procedures for Attention Deficit Disorders in Children," *Journal of Psychology and Christianity,* vol. 12, no. 4 (1993), pp. 357–74.

5. J. D. McKinney, M. Montague, and A. M. Horcutt, "Educational Assessment of Students With Attention Deficit Disorder," *Exceptional Children,* vol. 60, no. 2 (1993), pp. 125–31; M. Fowler, et al., *Ch.A.D.D. Educators Manual: An Indepth Look at Attention Deficit Disorders from an Educational Perspective* (Plantation, FL: CHADD, 1992).

6. EEG screenings and brain mappings seem to have limited value in clinical diagnosis of ADHD. B. B. Phillips, et al., "Electroencephalography in Childhood Conduct and Behavior Disorders," *Clinical Electroencephalography,* vol. 24, no. 1 (1993), pp. 25–30.

The consensus in the medical community seems to be that these advanced techniques may be premature for clinical use. P. Francies, "Dr. Trock Talks about Brain Mapping," *Update,* vol. 94, no. 1 (1994), p. 1. At worst (according to Dr. Gary Trock, pediatric neurologist in the Detroit area), such tests could be a waste of time and money, offering false hope to parents and adults.

7. E. A. Schaughency and J. Rothlind, "Assessment and Classification of Attention Deficit Hyperactivity Disorders," *School Psychology Review,* vol. 20, no. 2 (1991), p. 197.

8. Jerome M. Sattler, *Assessment of Children,* 3rd ed. (San Diego, CA: Jerome M. Sattler, 1988).

9. Leopold Bellak, *The Thematic Apperception Test, The Children's Apperception Test, and The Senior Apperception Technique in Clinical Use.* (New York: Grune and Stratton, 1986), pp. 215–18.

10. Barkley, "Diagnosis and Assessment."

Chapter Five: If It's Not ADHD, What Else Could It Be?

1. In a large sample of children and adolescents, researchers found that the highest comorbidity with ADHD was mild depression (77 percent), and the second highest was major depression (74 percent). Other conditions occurring less often (and in descending order) were oppositional defiant disorder and anxiety. J. Biederman, et al., "Psychiatric Comorbidity Among Referred Juveniles with Major Depression: Fact or Artifact?" *Journal of the American Academy of Child and Adolescent Psychiatry,* vol. 34 (1995), pp. 579–90. According to the American Psychiatric Association, *Diagnostic and Statistical Manual of Mental Disorders* (Washington, D.C.: American Psychiatric Association, 1995), or *DSM-IV*, the prevalence of Tourette's syndrome is four or five cases per 10,000 people.

2. J. R. Bemporad and K. W. Lee, "Affective Disorders," *Handbook of Clinical Assessment of Children and Adolescents,* vol. 2 (New York: New York University Press, 1988).

3. J. Biederman, et al., "Psychiatric Comorbidity"; R. Hunt, "Attention Deficit Disorder and Hyperactivity," *Handbook of Clinical Assessment of Children and Adolescents*; and Stephen P. McDermott, M.D., Thomas Spencer, M.D., and Timothy

E. Wilens, M.D., "Common Sense about Adult AD/HD" *Attention,* vol 2, no. 2 (Fall 1995), pp. 36–41.

4. A. E. Kazdin, "Childhood Depression," *Treatment of Childhood Disorders* (New York: Guilford Press, 1989), pp. 135–66.

5. R. A. Barkley, *Attention Deficit Hyperactivity Disorder; A Handbook for Diagnosis and Treatment* (New York: Guilford Press, 1990), pp. 191–96.

6. Ibid.

7. D. Comings, *Tourette's Syndrome and Human Behavior* (Duarte, CA: Hope Press, 1990); and E. R. Knell and D. E. Comings, "Tourette's Syndrome and Attention Deficit Hyperactivity Disorder: Evidence for a Genetic Relationship," *Journal of Clinical Psychiatry,* vol. 54 (1993), pp. 331–37.

8. Knell and Comings, "Tourette's Syndrome"; K. O. Yeates and R. A. Bornstein, "Attention Deficit Disorder and Neuropsychological Functioning in Children With Tourette's Syndrome," Neuropsychology, vol. 8, no. 1 (1994), pp. 65–74.

9. D. E. Comings and B. G. Comings, "Controlled Study of Tourette's Syndrome, Attention Deficit Disorder, Learning Disorders and School Problems," *American Journal of Human Genetics,* vol. 41 (1987), pp. 701–41; J. Sverd, K. D. Gadow, and L. M. Paolicelli, "Methylphenidate Treatment of Attention Deficit Hyperactivity Disorder in Boys with Tourette's Syndrome," *Journal of the American Academy of Child and Adolescent Psychiatry,* vol. 28 (1989), pp. 547–79; K. D. Gadow, E. E. Nolan, and J. Sverd, "Methylphenidate in Hyperactive Boys With Co-morbid Tic Disorder: II. Short-Term Behavior Effects in School Settings," *Journal of the American Academy of Child and Adolescent Psychiatry,* vol. 31 (1992), pp. 462–71.

10. S. Neuwirth, *Attention Deficit Hyperactivity Disorder: Decade of the Brain* (Washington D.C.: U.S. Government Printing Office, 1994); *DSM-IV*, pp. 92–93.

11. S. Goldstein, Ph.D., and M. Goldstein, M.D., *Managing Attention Disorders in Children* (New York: John Wiley, 1990), pp. 157–58; S. K. Shapiro and B. D. Garfinkel, "The Occurrence of Behavior Disorders in Children: The Interdependence of Attention Deficit Disorder and Behavior Disorders in Children," *Journal of the American Academy of Child Psychiatry,* vol. 25 (1986), pp. 809–19.

12. R. Schachar and R. Tannock, "A Test of Our Hypotheses for the Comorbidity of Attention Deficit Hyperactivity Disorder and Conduct Disorder," *Journal of the American Academy of Child and Adolescent Psychiatry,* vol. 34 (1995), pp. 639–48; H. A. Foley, O. C. Carlton, and R. J. Howell, "The Relationship of Attention Deficit Hyperactivity Disorder and Conduct Disorder to Juvenile Delinquency: Legal Implications," *Bulletin of the American Academy of Psychiatry and the Law,* vol. 24, no. 3 (1996), pp. 333–45; and R. Loeber et al., "Initiation, Escalation, and Desistence in Juvenile Offending and Their Correlates," *Journal of Criminal Law and Criminology,* vol. 82 (1991), pp. 36–82.

13. *DSM-IV.*

14. Barkley, *Attention Deficit Hyperactivity Disorder: A Clinical Workbook* (New York: Guilford Press, 1990), S. Goldstein and M. Goldstein, *Managing Attention Disorder in Children* (New York: John Wiley, 1990); G. J. August and B. D. Garfinkel, "Comorbidity of ADHD and Reading Disability Among Clinic-Referred Children," *Journal of Abnormal Child Psychology,* vol. 18 (1990), pp. 29–45; P. J. Frick and B. B. Lahey, "The Nature and Characteristics of Attention

Deficit Hyperactivity Disorder," *School Psychology Review,* vol. 20, no. 2 (1991), pp. 163–73.

Chapter Six: How to Treat ADHD

1. Edna D. Copeland, *Medications for Attention Disorders* (Atlanta: Resurgens Press, 1994), p. 163.

2. C. L. Carlson, et al., "Single and Combined Effects of Methylphenidate and Behavior Therapy on the Classroom Performance of Children with Attention Deficit-Hyperactivity Disorder," *Journal of Abnormal Child Psychology,* vol. 20, no. 2 (1992), pp. 213–32.

3. A. D. Anastopoulos, G. J. DuPaul, and R. A. Barkley, "Stimulant Medication and Parent-Training Therapies for Attention Deficit Hyperactivity Disorder," *Journal of Learning Disabilities,* vol. 24, no. 4 (1991), pp. 210–18.

4. John Taylor, *Helping Your Hyperactive/Attention Deficit Child* (Rocklin, CA: Prima Publishing, 1994), pp. 12–27.

5. Copeland, *Medications.*

6. Ibid., as well as numerous testimonials from patients, experts, and persons interviewed for this book.

7. Copeland, *Medications.*

8. R. L. Findling, "Open-Label Treatment of Comorbid Depression and Attentional Disorders. With Co-Administration of Serotonin Reuptake Inhibitors and Psychostimulants in Children, Adolescents, and Adults: A Case Study," *Journal of Child and Adolescent Psychopharmacology,* vol. 6 (Fall 1996), pp. 165–75; L. Barrickman et al., "Treatment of ADHD

with Fluoxetine: A Preliminary Trial," *Journal of the American Academy of Child and Adolescent Psychiatry,* vol. 30, no. 5 (1991), pp. 762–67; G. D. Gammon and T. E. Brown, "Fluoxetine and Methylphenidate in Combination for Treatment of Attention Deficit Disorder and Comorbid Depressive Disorder," *Journal of Child and Adolescent Psychopharmacology,* vol. 3, no. 1 (1993), pp. 1–10.

9. Ibid

10. Mary Fowler, *Maybe You Know My Kid* (New York: Birch Lane Press, 1994), p. 167.

11. Barbara Ingersoll, *Your Hyperactive Child* (New York: Doubleday, 1988), pp. 65–66; Fowler, *Maybe You Know My Kid;* Copeland, *Medications.*

12. T. P. Hoehn and A. A. Baumeister, "A Critique of the Application of Sensory Integration Therapy to Children with Learning Disabilities," *Journal of Learning Disabilities,* vol. 27 (1994), pp. 338–50.

13. Fowler, *Maybe You Know My Kid;* Martin Baren, M.D., "Managing ADHD," *Contemporary Pediatrics,* vol. 11 (December 1994), pp. 29–48; Paul H. Wender, M.D., *The Hyperactive Child, Adolescent and Adult* (New York: Oxford University Press, 1987), p. 73.

14. Stephen C. Copps, M.D., *The Attending Physician: Attention Deficit Disorder* (Atlanta: SPI Press, 1992), p. 59.

15. *Pediatrics in Review,* vol. 15, no. 1 (January 1994), p. 11. Timothy P. Culbert, G. A. Banez, and M. I. Reiff, "Children Who Have Attentional Disorders: Interventions," *Pediatrics in Review,* vol. 15, no. 1 (January 1994) p. 11.

Chapter Seven: Ritalin: The Facts

1. J. D. Lawrence, D. B. Lawrence, and D. S. Carson, "Optimizing ADHD Therapy with Sustained-Release Methylphenidate," *American Family Physician,* vol. 55, no. 5 (1997), pp. 1705–09; D. J. Safer and J. M. Krager, "A Survey of Medication Treatment for Hyperactive/Inattentive Students," *Journal of the American Medical Association,* vol. 260 (1988), pp. 2256–58.

2. Ibid. "In the United States, 90 percent of children with ADHD take methylphenidate. . . . Methylphenidate is most commonly chosen because of its proven safety and efficacy. . . . Methylphenidate is also favored because it has been associated for more than 40 years with positive outcomes (up to 79 percent response) in children with ADHD." (Lawrence, Lawrence, and Carson, 1997) W. E. Pelham, et al., "Sustained Release and Standard Methylphenidate Effects on Cognitive and Social Behavior in Children with Attention Deficit Disorder," *Pediatrics,* vol. 80 (1987), pp. 491–501. See also J. Elia, "Drug Treatment for Hyperactive Children: Therapeutic Guidelines," *Drugs,* vol. 46 (1993), pp. 863–71.

3. G. J. DuPaul and M. D. Rapport, "Does Methylphenidate Normalize the Classroom Performance of Children with Attention Deficit Disorder?" *Journal of the American Academy of Child and Adolescent Psychiatry,* vol. 32, no. 1 (1993), 190–98.

4. W. E. Pelham, et al., "Methylphenidate and Baseball Playing in ADHD Children: Who's on First?" *Journal of Consulting and Clinical Psychology,* vol. 58, no. 1 (1990), pp. 130–33.

5. R. G. Klein, "Clinical Efficacy of Methylphenidate in Children and Adolescents," *Encephale,* vol. 19, no. 2 (1993), pp. 89–93. The authors in one study point out that a deceleration of growth velocity is the only identified long-term side effect. It occurs only after more than one year of treatment at greater than low doses, and it appears completely reversible with treatment cessation. W. E. Pelham, et al., "Separate and Combined Effects of Methylphenidate and Behavior Modification on Boys with Attention Deficit Hyperactivity Disorder in the Classroom," *Journal of Consulting and Clinical Psychology,* vol. 61, no. 3 (1993), pp. 506–15.

6. Paul H. Wender, *The Hyperactive Child, Adolescent and Adult: Attention Deficit Disorder Through the Lifespan* (New York: Oxford University Press, 1987), p. 60.

7. Michael Lechner, "Attention Deficit Hyperactivity Disorder," *Clinical Update,* vol. 2, no. 4 (1995), pp. 1–6.

8. Dr. James Swanson was interviewed by telephone in April 1995.

9. B. B. Osman, "Coordinating Care in the Prescription and Use of Methylphenidate with Children," in L. L. Greenhill and B. B. Osman, eds., *Ritalin: Theory and Patient Management* (New York: Mary Ann Liebert, 1992).

10. J. E. Fried, "Use of Ritalin in the Practice of Pediatrics," in Greenhill and Osman, *Ritalin: Theory and Patient Management.*

11. J. M. Halperin, J. H. Newcorn, and V. Sharma, "Ritalin: Diagnostic Comorbidity and Attentional Measures," in Greenhill and Osman, *Ritalin: Theory and Patient Management;* Lawrence, Lawrence, and Carson, "Optimizing ADHD

Therapy"; and J. Elia and J. L. Rapoport, "Ritalin Versus Dextroamphetamine in ADHD: Both Should Be Tried," in Greenhill and Osman, *Ritalin: Theory and Patient Management.*

12. Edna D. Copeland, *Medications for Attention Disorders* (Atlanta: Resurgens Press, 1994), p. 177.

13. Ibid.

14. Fried, "Use of Ritalin."

15. R. A. Barkley, "Attention Deficit Hyperactivity Disorder," *Psychiatric Annals,* vol. 21, no. 12 (1991), pp. 725–33.

16. E. Tirosh et al., "Effect of Methylphenidate on Sleep in Children with Attention Deficit Hyperactivity Disorder: An Activity Monitor Study," *American Journal of Diseases of Children,* vol. 147, no. 12 (1993), pp. 1313–15.

17. R. A. Barkley, *Attention Deficit Hyperactivity Disorder: A Handbook of Diagnosis and Treatment* (New York: Guilford Press, 1990), p. 587. In "Medication Therapy," an article in Barkley's book, authors G. J. DuPaul and Barkley explain that children with ADHD frequently report these same symptoms, notably stomachaches and headaches, before taking medication and even when on a placebo.

18. "Attention Deficit Disorder—Part II," *Harvard Mental Health Letter,* vol. 11, no. 11 (May 1995), pp. 1–3.

19. Ibid.

20. S. C. Copps, *The Attending Physician: Attention Deficit Disorder* (Atlanta: SPI Press, 1992), p. 75.

21. Edna D. Copeland and Valerie L. Love, *Attention, Please!* (Atlanta: SPI Press, 1991), p. 142.

22. Barkley, op. cit. The author states that "heart rate variability is reduced by methylphenidate" and that "changes in cardiovascular functioning are considered mild."

23. Studies of methylphenidate show significant elevations of the resting heart rate in previously unmedicated children, but with continued drug treatment, only a minor increase is observed. Methylphenidate resulted in no consistent or clinically meaningful blood pressure changes, and no EKG irregularities. D. J. Safer, "Relative Cardiovascular Safety of Psychostimulants used to Treat Attention Deficit Hyperactivity Disorder," *Journal of Child and Adolescent Psychopharmacology,* vol. 2, no. 4 (1992), pp. 279–90.

24. Copeland and Love, *Attention, Please!*

25. P. S. Accardo, *Attention Deficit Disorders and Hyperactivity in Children* (New York: Marcel Dekker, 1991), p. 321.

26. *Physicians' Desk Reference* (Montvale, NJ: Medical Economics Company, 1997), or *PDR,* p. 867

27. Accardo, *Attention Deficit,* p. 322. V. Gross-Tsur and colleagues conclude that methylphenidate is effective in treating even children with epilepsy and ADHD, and it is safe in ADHD children who are seizure-free. V. Gross-Tsur, et al., "Epilepsy and Attention Deficit Hyperactivity Disorder: Is Methylphenidate Safe and Effective?" *Journal of Pediatrics,* vol. 130 (1997), pp. 40–44.

28. Accardo, *Attention Deficit,* p. 321.

29. *PDR,* p. 867.

30. These newspaper reports are discussed in Chapter 1.

31. R. A. Barkley, "Predicting the Response of Hyperkinetic Children to Stimulant Drugs: A Review," *Journal of*

Abnormal Child Psychology, vol. 4 (1976), pp. 327–48; and L. J. Barin, *A Parent's Guide to Attention Deficit Disorders* (New York: Dell, 1991), p. 12.

32. Dr. Arthur Robin was interviewed in March 1995.

33. Martin Baren, M.D., "The Case for Ritalin: A Fresh Look at the Controversy," *Contemporary Pediatrics,* vol. 6, (January 1989), pp. 16–28.

34. A. S. Bloom and colleagues describe the case of one six-year-old boy who developed a psychotic disturbance while in methylphenidate therapy. A. S. Bloom, et al., "Methylphenidate—Induced Delusional Disorder in a Child with Attention Deficit Disorder with Hyperactivity," *Journal of the American Academy of Child and Adolescent Psychiatry,* vol. 27, no. 1 (1988), pp. 88–89. Y. Mino and colleagues tell of a 16-year-old girl who had an acute psychotic reaction associated with methylphenidate treatment. Y. Mino, et al., "Methylphenidate Psychosis in an Adolescent with Attention Deficit Disorder," *Japanese Journal of Child and Adolescent Psychiatry,* vol. 27, no. 3 (1986), pp. 178–87.

35. Peter Breggin, M.D., *Toxic Psychiatry* (New York: St. Martin's Press, 1991), p. 277.

36. Peter Breggin, M.D., *Talking Back to Ritalin: What Doctors Aren't Telling You About Stimulants for Children* (Monroe, ME: Common Courage Press, 1998).

37. N. D. Volkow et al., "Is Methylphenidate like Cocaine? Studies on Their Pharmacokinetics and Distribution in the Human Brain," *Archives of General Psychiatry,* vol. 52 (1995), pp. 456–63; B. B. Osman, "Coordinating Care in the Prescription and Use of Methylphenidate with Chil-

dren," in L. L. Greenhill and B. B. Osman, eds., *Ritalin: Theory and Patient Management,* (New York: Mary Ann Liebert, 1992), p. 123; P. Kennedy, L. Terdal, and L. Fusetti, *The Hyperactive Child Book* (New York: St. Martin's Press, 1993), p. 58.

38. N. D. Volkow et al., "Is Methylphenidate Like Cocaine? Studies on Their Pharmacokinetics and Distribution in the Human Brain," *Archives of General Psychiatry,* vol. 52 (1995), pp. 456–63.

39. J. Biederman, et al., "Psychoactive Substance Use Disorders in Adults with Attention Deficit Hyperactivity Disorder: Effects of ADHD and Psychiatric Comorbidity," *American Journal of Psychiatry,* vol. 152 (1995), pp. 281–302; M. T. Lyndskey and D. M. Gergusson, "Childhood Conduct Problems, Attention Deficit Behaviors, and Adolescent Alcohol, Tobacco, and Illicit Drug Use," *Journal of Abnormal Child Psychology,* vol. 23 (1995), pp. 281–302.

40. J. A. Halikas, et al., "Predicting Substance Abuse in Juvenile Offenders: Attention Deficit Disorder vs. Aggressivity," *Child Psychiatry and Human Development,* vol. 21, no. 1 (1990), pp. 49–55. This idea of a link between aggression and ADHD was first proposed in J. Looney, "Substance Abuse in Adolescents: Diagnostic Issues Derived from Studies of Attention Deficit Disorder with Hyperactivity," *National Institute on Drug Abuse: Research Monograph Series,* vol. 77 (1988), pp. 19–26.

41. A study conducted at Massachusetts General Hospital in Boston followed 140 children for four years beginning at ages ranging from 10 to 13. It was reported in the January 1997 of the *Journal of the American Academy of Child and*

Adolescent Psychiatry and summarized in D. Mann, "ADHD May Make Kids More Prone to Drug Abuse," *Medical Tribune News Service* (January 6, 1997), p. 1.

42. "Q&A: An Interview with John Werry, M.D.," *Attention!* (CHADD publication) (Summer 1995), p. 30.

43. D. L. Wodrich, *Attention Deficit Hyperactivity Disorder* (Baltimore: Paul H. Brooks, 1994), p. 173.

44. D. Safer, R. Allen, and E. Barr, "Depression of Growth in Hyperactive Children on Stimulant Drugs," *New England Journal of Medicine,* vol. 287 (1972), pp. 217–20.

45. B. McNutt, J. Ballard, and R. Boileau, "The Effects of Long-Term Stimulant Medication on Growth and Body Composition of Hyperactive Children," *Psychopharmacology Bulletin,* vol. 12 (1976), pp. 13–14; M. K. Dulcan, "Attention Deficit Disorder: Evaluation and Treatment," *Pediatric Annals,* vol. 14, no. 5 (1985), pp. 383–98; J. E. Fried, "Use of Ritalin"; T. J. Spencer, et al., "Growth Deficits in ADHD Children Revised: Evidence for Disorder-Associated Growth Delays?" *Journal of the American Academy of Child and Adolescent Psychiatry,* vol. 35, no. 11 (1996), pp. 1460–69.

46. Spencer et al., "Growth Deficits."

47. Copeland, *Medications,* p. 180.

48. "Toxicology and Carcinogenesis Studies of Methylphenidate Hydrochloride (CASE No. 298-59-9) in F344/N Rates and B6C3F Mice (Feed Studies)," National Toxicology Program, TR-439, *Federal Register,* vol. 1, no. 85 (May 1, 1996), pp. 19306–307.

49. B. Hendrick, "HealthWatch: Government's Ritalin Alert Not Needed, Some Experts Say," *Atlanta Journal and*

Constitution (January 24, 1996), p. D3. The article quotes Dr. Alan J. Zametkin, Dr. Theodore Atkinson, Dr. Julie B. Schweitzer, and R. Ann Abramovitz.

50. According to Dr. Murray Lumpkin, the FDA's deputy drug director, "We felt physicians and parents should know this and have a right to know this." He added, "But it's not enough of a signal that we think kids should be taken off the drug." The FDA also ordered Ciba-Geigy, then the manufacturer of Ritalin, to add the mouse findings to the drug's label and notify doctors about the potential risk. See "Drug Cancer Link Probed," Associated Press, *Newsday* (January 13, 1996), p. A11.

51. Hendrick, "HealthWatch."

52. D. McLearn, "Ritalin Studies," FDA press release (January 12, 1996), p. 1.

53. In 1992 Robert Diener, a toxicologist for Ciba-Geigy, revealed, perhaps for the first time to the public, some of the early research conducted by Ciba-Geigy on methylphenidate that was previously available to the FDA only in Ciba-Geigy's New Drug Application for Ritalin in the 1950s. Essentially, toxicology studies on rats, mice, and dogs found no evidence of liver cancer or any other kind of cancer, even when megadoses of methylphenidate were given over prolonged periods. R. M. Diener, "Toxicology of Ritalin," in Greenhill and Osman, *Ritalin Theory and Patient Management,* pp. 35–43.

54. McLearn, "Ritalin Studies."

55. Copeland, *Medications,* p. 173

56. Ibid.

57. T. W. Phelan, *All About Attention Deficit Disorder* (Glen Ellyn, IL: CMI, 1993), p. 166.

58. Accardo, *Attention Deficit,* p. 308.

59. J. D. Kent and colleagues found that children with ADHD derive substantial symptom reduction from Ritalin administered in the late afternoon. There was no adverse effect on the sleep of the twelve children in this study. J. D. Kent et al., "Effects of Late-Afternoon Methylphenidate Administration on Behavior and Sleep in Attention Deficit Hyperactivity Disorder," *Pediatrics,* vol. 96, no. 2 (1995), pp. 320–25.

60. *PDR,* p. 867; W. J. Bailey, "Factline on Non-Medical Use of Ritalin (Methylphenidate)," Indiana Prevention Resource Center, *Factline,* no. 9 (November 1995), pp. 1–4.

61. S. C. Copps, *The Attending Physician: Attention Deficit Disorder* (Atlanta: SPI Press, 1992), pp. 67–68.

62. W. Pelham, et al., "Sustained Release and Standard Methylphenidate Effects on Cognitive and Social Behavior in Children with Attention Deficit Disorder," *Pediatrics,* vol. 4 (1987), pp. 491–501; B. Birmaher, et al., "Sustained Release Methylphenidate: Pharmacokinetic Studies in ADHD Males," *Journal of the American Academy of Child and Adolescent Psychiatry,* vol. 28 (1989), pp. 768–72; P. A. Fitzpatrick, et al., "Effects of Sustained-Release and Standard Preparations of Methylphenidate on Attention Deficit Disorder," *Journal of the American Academy of Child and Adolescent Psychiatry,* vol. 31 (1992), pp. 226–34.

63. J. D. Lawrence, D. B. Lawrence, and D. S. Carson, "Optimizing ADHD Therapy with Sustained-Release Methylphenidate," *American Family Physician,* vol. 55, no. 5 (1997), pp. 1705–09.

64. Fitzpatrick, et al., "Effects of Sustained Release"; Lawrence, Lawrence, and Carson, "Optimizing ADHD."

65. *PDR,* p. 866; Bailey, "Factline on Non-Medical Use."

66. Karen Thomas, "Ritalin Maker's Ties to Advocates Probed," *USA Today* (November 16, 1995).

67. Volkow, et al., "Is Methylphenidate Like Cocaine?"

68. "For a physician to prescribe Ritalin or any drug and not provide for follow-up is a disservice to parents and children, which borders on malpractice." Osman, "Coordinating Care," p. 123.

69. R. A. Barkley, *Attention Deficit Hyperactivity Disorder: A Handbook for Diagnosis and Treatment* (New York: Guilford Press, 1990), p. 593.

70. Kennedy, Terdal, and Fusetti, *Hyperactive Child Book,* p. 53.

71. S. B. Campbell, "Hyperactivity in Preschoolers: Correlates and Prognostic Implications," *Clinical Psychology Review,* vol. 5 (1985), pp. 405–28.

72. *PDR,* p. 866.

73. Ibid.

74. K. D. Gadow and colleagues contend that there is no evidence that methylphenidate alters the severity of a tic disorder, but it may have a weak effect on the frequency of motor tics by increasing them and a weak effect on verbal tics by decreasing them. In general, they conclude, Ritalin is a safe and effective treatment for ADHD children who also have a tic disorder. K. D. Gadow et al., "Efficacy of Methylphenidate for Attention Deficit Hyperactivity Disorder in Children with Tic Disorder," *Archives of General Psychiatry,* vol. 52, no. 6 (1995), pp. 445–55.

75. The only research available comes from the New Drug Application research information from Ciba-Geigy, in Diener, "Toxicology of Ritalin." Diener indicates that all studies with animals from pregnancy to lactation indicate no adverse effects on embryos or the young animals.

Chapter Eight: Ritalin Do's and Don'ts

1. B. B. Osman, "Coordinating Care in the Prescription and Use of Methylphenidate with Children," in L. L. Greenhill and B. B. Osman, eds., *Ritalin: Theory and Patient Management* (New York: Mary Ann Liebert, 1992), pp. 123–26.

2. J. Elia and J. L. Rapoport, "Ritalin Versus Dextroamphetamine in ADHD: Both Should Be Tried," in Greenhill and Osman, *Ritalin: Theory and Patient Management,* p. 71.

3. M. K. Dulcan, "Attention Deficit Disorder: Evaluation and Treatment," *Pediatric Annals,* vol. 14, no. 5 (1985), p. 388; and G. J. DuPaul and R. A. Barkley, "Medication Therapy," in R. A. Barkley, *Attention Deficit Hyperactivity Disorder: A Handbook for Diagnosis and Treatment* (New York: Guilford Press, 1990), p. 589.

4. R. A. Barkley, "Diagnosis and Assessment of Attention Deficit Hyperactivity Disorder," *Comprehensive Mental Health Care,* vol. 1, no. 1 (1991), pp. 27–32.

5. American Academy of Family Physicians, "How to Take Medicine for ADHD," patient information handout, *American Family Physician,* vol. 55, no. 5 (1997).

6. *Physician's Desk Reference,* (Montvale, NJ: Medical Economics Data Production Company, 1997), p. 867.

7. J. E. Fried, "Use of Ritalin in the Practice of Pediatrics," in Goodhill and Osman, *Ritalin: Theory and Patient Management*, p. 137.

8. A. L. Robin, "Training Families with ADHD Adolescents," in R. A. Barkley, *Attention Deficit Hyperactivity Disorder: A Handbook for Diagnosis and Treatment* (New York: Guilford Press, 1990), pp. 474–75.

9. According to R. G. Klein, "None of the studies has found that children on stimulants were less spontaneous with adults than children who were not hyperactive." R. G. Klein, "An Update on the Stimulant Treatment of ADHD," *CHADDer,* (Spring/Summer 1992), p. 19. C. K. Whalen and associates found that children on Ritalin were more often described by peers as being cooperative and fun to be around. C. K. Whalen, et al., "Does Stimulant Medication Improve the Peer Status of Hyperactive Children?" *Journal of Consulting and Clinical Psychology,* vol. 57, no. 4 (1989), pp. 545–49. M. K. Walker and colleagues found that after treatment with Ritalin, children were judged to be less angry and hostile. M. K. Walker, et al., "Effects of Methylphenidate Hydrochloride on the Subjective Reporting of Mood in Children with Attention Deficit Disorder," *Issues in Mental Health Nursing,* vol. 9, no. 4 (1988), pp. 373–85. R. Klorman and colleagues found that one treatment effect was that adolescents rated themselves as having an elevated mood while taking methylphenidate. R. Klorman, et al., "Clinical Effects of a Controlled Study of Methylphenidate on Adolescents with Attention Deficit Disorder," *Journal of the American Academy of Child and Adolescent Psychiatry,* vol. 29, no. 5 (1990), pp. 702–09.

10. A. L. Robin was interviewed in May 1995.

11. D. P. Cantwell, "Psychopharmacologic Treatment of ADHD: Non-Stimulant Medications," *CHADDer* (Spring/

Summer 1990), p. 8; A. F. Schatzberg and J. O. Cole, *Manual of Clinical Psychopharmacology,* 2nd ed. (Washington, D.C.: American Psychiatric Press, 1991), pp. 252–53; and R. D. Hunt, S. Lau, and J. Ryu, "Alternative Therapies for ADHD," in Greenhill and Osman, *Ritalin: Theory and Patient Management,* pp. 75–95.

Chapter Nine: Other Medications for ADHD

1. D. P. Cantwell, "Psychopharmacologic Treatment of ADHD: Non-Stimulant Medications," *CHADDer* (Spring/ Summer 1990), p. 8; A. F. Schatzberg and J. O. Cole, *Manual of Clinical Psychopharmacology,* 2nd ed. (Washington, D.C.: American Psychiatric Press, 1991), pp. 252–53; and R. D. Hunt, S. Lau, and J. Ryu, "Alternative Therapies for ADHD," in L. L. Greenhill and B. B. Osman, eds., *Ritalin: Theory and Patient Management* (New York: Mary Ann Liebert, 1992), pp. 75–95.

2. G. J. DuPaul and R. A. Barkley, "Medication Therapy," in R. A. Barkley, *Attention Deficit Hyperactivity Disorder: A Handbook for Diagnosis and Treatment* (New York: Guilford Press, 1990), pp. 573–612; and Hunt, Lau, and Ryu, "Alternative Therapies for ADHD," pp. 75–95.

3. DuPaul and Barkley, "Medication Therapy," p. 589. The authors state: "There are no reported cases of addiction or serious drug dependence to date with these [methylphenidate] medications."

4. S. R. Pliska, "Attention Deficit Hyperactivity Disorder: A Clinical Review," *American Family Physician,* vol. 43, no. 4 (1991), pp. 1267–75.

5. Edna D. Copeland, *Medications for Attention Disorders* (Atlanta: Resurgens Press, 1994), pp. 161–206.

6. *Physician's Desk Reference,* (Montvale, NJ: Medical Economics Company, 1997), p. 2210.

7. Ibid., p. 2210.

8. Ibid., p. 2210.

9. Copeland, *Medications,* p. 197.

10. J. D. Lawrence, D. B. Lawrence, and D. S. Carson, "Optimizing ADHD Therapy with Sustained-Release Methylphenidate," *American Family Physician,* vol. 55, no. 5 (1997), pp. 1705–06.

11. K. Calis, D. Brother, and J. Elia, "Therapy Reviews: Attention Deficit Hyperactivity Disorder," *Clinical Pharmacy,* vol. 9 (1990), pp. 632–42; and Copeland, *Medications,* p. 199.

12. Abbott Laboratories, drug insert sheet, "Cylert (Pemoline)," September 1991. The insert says: "Safety and effectiveness in children below the age of 6 years have not been established."

13. T. E. Wilens and J. Biederman, "The Stimulants," *Psychiatric Clinics of North America,* vol. 15, no. 1 (1992), pp. 191–222. The authors state that children prescribed Cylert should be monitored for chemical hepatitis. See also Copeland, *Medications,* p. 183; and T. P. Culbert, G. A. Banex, and M. Reiff, "Children Who Have Attention Disorders: Interventions," *Pediatrics in Review,* vol. 15 (1994), pp. 5–14.

14. J. Elia and J. L. Rapoport, "Ritalin Versus Dextroamphetamine in ADHD: Both Should Be Tried," in Greenhill

and Osman, *Ritalin: Theory and Patient Management,* pp. 69–74; and Lawrence, Lawrence, and Carson, "Optimizing ADHD Therapy," pp. 1705–09.

15. Sam Goldstein, Ph.D., and Michael Goldstein, M.D., *Managing Attention Disorders in Children* (New York: John Wiley, 1990), p. 246; see also *PDR*, p. 2649.

16. Stephen C. Copps, M.D., *The Attending Physician: Attention Deficit Disorder* (Atlanta: SPI Press, 1992), p. 69.

17. *PDR,* p. 2649.

18. Ibid.; and Copeland, *Medications,* p. 193.

19. *PDR,* p. 2649.

20. Cantwell, "Psychopharmacologic Treatment of ADHD," pp. 8–9; and Hunt, Lau, and Ryu, "Alternative Therapies for ADHD," pp. 75–80.

21. Hunt, Lau, and Ryu, "Alternative Therapies for ADHD," pp. 75–80.

22. Ibid.; and J. Biederman, et al., "A Double-Blind Placebo Controlled Study of Desipramine in the Treatment of ADHD," *Journal of the American Academy of Child and Adolescent Psychiatry,* vol. 28, no. 5 (1989), pp. 777–84.

23. According to Russell Barkley, the coexistence of ADHD with other behavioral and emotional disorders is "generally quite common with up to 44% having at least one other psychiatric disorder." Over half of ADHD children have significant problems in social relationships with other children. R. A. Barkley, "Attention Deficit Hyperactivity Disorder," *Psychiatric Annals,* vol. 21, no. 12 (1991), p. 730. Barkley and colleagues state that 40 percent of ADHD chil-

dren and 65 percent of ADHD adolescents have opposi-
tional defiant disorder. R. A. Barkley, G. J. DuPaul, and
M. B. McMurray, "A Comprehensive Evaluation of Atten-
tion Deficit Disorder With and Without Hyperactivity as
Defined by Research Criteria," *Journal of Consulting and
Clinical Psychology,* vol. 58 (1990), pp. 775–89.

24. J. Biederman, et al., "Family Genetic and Psychosocial
Risk Factors in Clinically Referred Children and Adolescents with *DSM-III* Attention Deficit Disorder," unpublished ms., Massachusetts General Hospital, Boston, 1989.
See also J. Biederman, K. Munir, and D. Knee, "Conduct
and Oppositional Disorder in Clinically Referred Children
with Attention Deficit Disorder: A Controlled Family Study,"
*Journal of the American Academy of Child and Adolescent Psy-
chiatry,* vol. 26 (1987), pp. 724–27.

25. A. F. Schatzberg and J. O. Cole, *Manual of Clinical
Psychopharmacology,* 2nd ed. (Washington, D.C.: American
Psychiatric Press, 1991), p. 256; and Hunt, Lau, and Ryu,
"Alternative Therapies for ADHD," pp. 75–80.

26. Hunt, Lau, and Ryu, "Alternative Therapies for ADHD,"
pp. 75–80; Biederman et al., "A Double-Blind Placebo";
and M. A. Riddle, et al., "Desipramine Treatment of Boys
with Attention Deficit Hyperactivity Disorder and Tics:
Preliminary Clinical Experience," *Journal of the American
Academy of Child and Adolescent Psychiatry,* vol. 27, no. 6
(1988), pp. 811–14.

27. Sam Goldstein, Ph.D., and Michael Goldstein, M.D.,
Managing Attention Disorders in Children (New York: John
Wiley, 1990), p. 253.

28. Copeland, *Medications,* p. 226.

29. Ibid.

30. Ibid.

31. *PDR,* p. 937.

32. Copeland, *Medications,* p. 208.

33. S. R. Pliska, "Tricyclic Antidepressants in the Treatment of Children with Attention Deficit Disorder," *Journal of the American Academy of Child and Adolescent Psychiatry,* vol. 26, no. 2 (1987), pp. 127–32.

34. *PDR,* p. 875.

35. Copeland, *Medications,* p. 216.

36. *PDR,* p. 875.

37. Ibid.

38. Cantwell, "Psychopharmacologic Treatment of ADHD," pp. 8–9; and Hunt, Lau, and Ryu, "Alternative Therapies for ADHD," pp. 75–80.

39. *PDR,* p. 1178.

40. Hunt, Lau, and Ryu, "Alternative Therapies for ADHD," pp. 80–88; and Timothy P. Culbert, M.D., Gerard A. Banez, Ph.D., and Michael I. Reiff, M.D., "Children Who Have Attention Disorders: Interventions," *Pediatrics in Review,* vol. 15, no. 1 (January 1994), pp. 5–14.

41. Hunt, Lau, and Ryu, "Alternative Therapies for ADHD," pp. 75–80.

42. Ibid.

43. Ibid.

44. Ibid.

45. D. M. Ross and S. A. Ross, *Hyperactivity: Current Issues, Research, and Theory,* 2nd ed. (New York: John Wiley, 1984).

46. "Two Pharmacologic Agents Show ADHD Promise," *Primary Psychiatry* (March 1996), pp. 14–15; *Pediatric News* (March 1995), p. 2. K. A. Batoosingh, "Scoping Available Drugs for ADHD Alternative," *Pediatric News* (March 1995), p. 2.

Chapter Ten: Psychological Treatment, Parent Training, and Support Groups

1. S. Neuwirth, *Attention Deficit Hyperactivity Disorder: Decade of the Brain,* National Institute of Mental Health publication no. 94-3572 (Washington, D.C.: U.S. Government Printing Office, 1994), p. 13.

2. H. Abikoff, "Interaction of Ritalin and Multimodal Therapy in the Treatment of Attention Deficit Hyperactive Behavior Disorder," in L. L. Greenhill and B. B. Osman, eds., *Ritalin: Theory and Patient Management* (New York: Mary Ann Liebert, 1992), pp. 147–54; J. H. Satterfield, D. P. Cantwell, and B. T. Satterfield, "Multimodality Treatment: A One Year Follow-Up of 84 Hyperactive Boys," *Archives of General Psychiatry,* vol. 36 (1979), pp. 965–74; A. D. Anastopoulos, G. J. DuPaul, and R. A. Barkley, "Stimulant Medication and Parent Training Therapies for Attention Deficit Hyperactivity Disorder," *Journal of Learning Disabilities,* vol. 24, no. 4 (1991), pp. 210–18; and G. J. DuPaul and R. A. Barkley, "Behavioral Contributions to Pharmacotherapy: The Utility of Behavioral Methodology in Medication Treatment of Children with Attention

Deficit Hyperactivity Disorder," *Behavior Therapy,* vol. 24, no. 1 (1993), pp. 47–65.

3. S. Goldstein, "Young Children at Risk: The Early Signs of Attention Deficit Hyperactivity Disorder," *CHADDer Box* (January 1991), p. 7.

4. M. C. Gridley, *Making Psychotherapy Work for You* (Waterford, MI: Minerva Press, 1988), pp. 2–5.

5. L. S. Coker and B. A. Thyer, "School- and Family-Based Treatment of Children with Attention Deficit Hyperactivity Disorder," *Families in Society,* vol. 71, no. 5 (1990), pp. 276–82.

6. J. Lock, "Developmental Considerations in the Treatment of School-Age Boys with ADHD: An Example of a Group Treatment Approach." *Journal of the American Academy of Child and Adolescent Psychiatry,* vol. 35, no. 11 (1996), pp. 1557–59; L. Braswell, "Cognitive-Behavioral Groups for Children Manifesting ADHD and Other Disruptive Behavior Disorders," *Special Services in the School,* vol. 8, no. 1 (1993), pp. 91–117. The author reviews outcome literature and concludes that there is considerable justification for using groups with ADHD children.

7. W. E. Pelham, et al., "Behavioral and Stimulant Treatment of Hyperactive Children: A Therapy Study with Methylphenidate Probes in a Within Subject Design," *Journal of Applied Behavior Analysis,* vol. 13 (1980), pp. 221–36; W. E. Pelham et al., "The Combination of Behavior Therapy and Methylphenidate in the Treatment of Attention Deficit Disorders: A Therapy Outcome Study," in J. Swanson and L. Bloomingdale, eds., *Attention Deficit Disorders,* vol. 4 (New York: Pergamon Press, 1990).

8. R. Hunt, "Attention Deficit Hyperactivity Disorder," in C. J. Kestenbaum and D. T. Williams, *Handbook of Clinical Assessment of Children and Adolescents,* vol. 11 (New York: New York University Press, 1988), p. 543.

9. R. A. Barkley, "What is the Role of Group Parent Training in the Treatment of ADD Children?" *Journal of Children in Contemporary Society,* vol. 19, no. 1 (1986), pp. 143–51; A. D. Anastopoulos et al., "Parent Training for Attention Deficit Hyperactivity Disorder: Its Impact on Parent Functioning," *Journal of Abnormal Child Psychology,* vol. 21, no. 5 (1993), pp. 581–96.

10. S. Pisterman, et al., "The Role of Parent Training in Treatment of Preschoolers with ADHD," *American Journal of Orthopsychiatry,* vol. 62, no. 3 (1992), pp. 397–408.

11. Anastopoulos, et al., "Parent Training."

12. For information about Children and Adults with Attention Deficit Disorders, see the Resources section of this book.

Chapter Eleven: Parenting the ADHD Child

1. M. Fisher, "Parenting Stress and the Child with Attention Deficit Hyperactivity Disorder," *Journal of Clinical Child Psychology,* vol. 19, no. 4 (1990), p. 337.

2. M. F. Breen and R. A. Barkley, "Child Psychopathology and Parenting Stress in Girls and Boys Having Attention Deficit Disorder with Hyperactivity," *Journal of Pediatric Psychology,* vol. 13 (1988), pp. 265–80.

3. C. Gilberg, G. Carlstrom, and P. Rasmussen, "Hyperkinetic Disorders in Seven-Year-Old Children with Perceptual, Motor and Attention Deficits," *Journal of Child Psychology,* vol. 24 (1983), pp. 233–46.

4. M. S. Befera and R. A. Barkley, "Hyperactive and Normal Girls and Boys: Mother-Child Interaction, Parent Psychiatric Status, and Child Psychopathology," *Journal of Child Psychology and Psychiatry,* vol. 26 (1985), pp. 439–52.

5. Fischer, "Parenting Stress," pp. 337–40.

6. "Attention Deficit Disorder— Part II," *Harvard Mental Health Letter* (May 1995), p. 2.

7. L. S. Cousins and G. Weiss, "Parent Training and Social Skills Training for Children with Attention Deficit Hyperactivity Disorder: How Can They Be Combined for Greater Effectiveness?" *Canadian Journal of Psychiatry,* vol. 38, no. 6 (1993), pp. 449–57; R. F. Newby, M. Fischer, and M. A. Roman, "Parent Training for Families with Children with ADHA," *School Psychology Review,* vol. 20, no. 2 (1991), pp. 252–65.

8. R. Forehand and R. McMahon, *Helping the Noncompliant Child: A Clinician's Guide to Parent Training* (New York: Guilford Press, 1981); A. D. Anastopoulos and R. A. Barkley, "Counseling and Training Parents," in R. A. Barkley, *Attention Deficit Hyperactivity Disorder: A Handbook for Diagnosis and Treatment* (New York: Guilford Press, 1990), pp. 397–431.

9. J. McCord, "Questioning the Value of Punishment," *Social Problems,* vol. 38, no. 2 (1991), pp. 167–79.

10. Z. Strassberg, et al., "Spanking in the Home and Children's Subsequent Aggression Towards Kindergarten Peers," *Development and Psychopathology,* vol. 6 (1994), pp.

445–61; M. A. Straus and G. K. Kantor, "Corporal Punishment of Adolescents by Parents: A Risk Factor in the Epidemiology of Depression, Suicide, Alcohol Abuse, Child Abuse, and Wife Beating," *Adolescence,* vol. 29, no. 115 (1994), pp. 543–61; M. A. Straus and D. A. Donnelly, *Beating the Devil Out of Them: Corporal Punishment in American Families* (New York: Lexington Books, 1994), pp. 149–69.

11. G. F. Koeske and R. D. Koeske, "The Buffering Effect of Social Support on Parental Stress," *American Journal of Orthopsychiatry,* vol. 60, no. 3 (1990), pp. 440–42.

12. There are several sites on the Internet for parents who would like to talk online with other parents about related ADHD issues.

Chapter Twelve: Educational Interventions

1. R. A. Barkley, "Attention Deficit Hyperactivity Disorder," *Psychiatric Annals,* vol. 21, no. 12 (1991), p. 725.

2. Ibid.

3. T. M. Black, *Straight Talk About American Education* (New York: Harcourt Brace Jovanovich, 1982).

4. Distributed by CHADD (see Resources).

5. L. J. Bain, *A Parent's Guide to Attention Deficit Disorders* (New York: Dell, 1991), p. 136–37.

6. L. J. Pfiffner and R. A. Barkley, "Educational Placement and Classroom Management," in R. A. Barkley, *Attention Deficit Hyperactivity Disorder: A Handbook for Diagnosis and Treatment* (New York: Guilford Press, 1990), pp. 508–09.

7. Barkley, "Attention Deficit."

8. T. L. Shelton and C. Crosswaite, "Prevention and Treatment Program for Kindergarten Students with ADHD," *CHADDer,* vol. 6, no. 1 (1992), pp. 16–33; and M. D. Rapport, "The Classroom Functioning and Treatment of Children with ADHD: Facts and Fictions," *CHADDer,* vol. 3, no. 2 (1989), pp. 4–5.

9. Barkley, "Attention Deficit."

10. Michael Merz was interviewed in 1995.

Chapter Thirteen: Adults with ADHD

1. H. C. Parker, "CH.A.D.D. Education Position Paper," *CHADDer,* vol. 4, no. 1 (1990), p. 21; J. J. Ratey, "Paying Attention to Attention in Adults," *CHADDer,* vol. 5, no. 2 (Fall/Winter 1991), pp. 13–14; and R. L. Findling, et al., "Venlafaxine in Adults with Attention Deficit Hyperactivity Disorder: An Open Clinical Trial," *Journal of Clinical Psychiatry,* vol. 57, no. 5 (1996), p. 184.

2. D. J. Morrow, "More Adults Diagnosed With Attention Deficit Disorder," *New York Times* (September 1, 1997).

3. W. O. Shekim, "Adult Attention Deficit Hyperactivity Disorder, Residual State (ADHD,RS)," *CH.A.D.D. Special Edition,* vol. 6, no. 3 (1992), p. 7; and P. H. Wender, *The Hyperactive Child, Adolescent, and Adult: Attention Deficit Disorder Through the Lifespan* (New York: Oxford University Press, 1987), p. 121.

4. Shekim, "Adult Attention Deficit."

5. P. H. Wender, D. R. Wood, and F. W. Reimherr, "Pharmacological Treatment of Attention Deficit Disorder, Residual Type (ADD-RT) in Adults," in L. L. Greenhill and B. B. Osman, eds., *Ritalin: Theory and Patient Management* (New York: Mary Ann Liebert, 1992), pp. 25–33; and J. J. Ratey, E. M. Hallowell, and C. L. Leveroni, "Pharmacotherapy for ADHD in Adults," Adult ADD Association, unpublished manuscript (n.d.), pp. 1–4.

6. T. Spencer et al., "A Double-Blind Crossover Comparison of Methylphenidate and Placebo in Adults with Childhood-Onset Attention Deficit Hyperactivity Disorder," *Archives of General Psychiatry,* vol. 52 (1995), pp. 434–43; and T. Wilens, et al., "A Systematic Assessment of Tricyclic Antidepressants in the Treatment of Adult Attention Deficit Hyperactivity Disorder," *Journal of Nervous and Mental Disorders,* vol. 183 (1995), pp. 48–50.

BIBLIOGRAPHY

Bain, Lisa J. *A Parent's Guide to Attention Deficit Disorders.* New York: Dell, 1991.

Barkley, R. A. *Attention Deficit Hyperactivity Disorder: A Handbook for Diagnosis and Treatment.* New York: Guilford Press, 1990.

Copeland, Edna D. *Medications for Attention Deficit Disorders and Related Medical Problems: A Comprehensive Handbook.* Atlanta, GA: SPI Press, 1991.

Copeland, Edna D., and Valerie L. Love. *Attention, Please!* Atlanta, GA: SPI Press, 1991.

Fowler, M. *Maybe You Know My Kid.* New York: Birch Lane Publishing, 1994.

Friedman, Ronald, and Guy Doyal. *Management of Children and Adolescents with Attention Deficit Hyperactivity Disorder.* Austin, TX: Pro-Ed, 1992.

Gordon, M. *ADHD/Hyperactivity: A Consumers Guide.* New York: GSI Publications, 1991.

Greenberg, G. S., and W. F. Horn. *Attention Deficit Hyperactivity Disorder: Questions and Answers for Parents.* Champaign, IL: Research Press, 1991.

Hallowell, Edward M., and John G. Ratey. *Answers to Distraction.* New York: Pantheon Books, 1995.

————. *Driven to Distraction.* New York: Pantheon Books, 1994.

Ingersol, B., and S. Goldstein. *Attention Deficit Disorder and Learning Disabilities: Realities, Myths, and Controversial Treatments.* New York: Doubleday, 1993.

Javorsky, James. *Alphabet Soup: A Recipe for Understanding and Treating Attention Deficit Hyperactivity Disorder.* Bloomfield Hills, MI: Minerva Press, 1993.

Johnson, Mary Jane. *ADD, a Lifetime Challenge.* Toledo: ADDult Support Network, 1993.

Kelly, Kate, and Peggy Ramundo. *You Mean I'm Not Lazy, Stupid or Crazy?* Cincinnati: Tyrell & Jenem Press, 1993.

Kennedy, Patricia, and Lydia Fusetti. *The Hyperactive Child Book.* New York: St. Martin's Press, 1993.

McCarney, S., and A. M. Bauer. *The Parents Guide to Attention Deficit Disorders.* Columbia, MO: Hawthorne Educational Services, 1990.

Shaya, James, and J. Windell. *Coping With Your Attention Deficit Disorder Child: A Practical Guide for Management.* Bloomfield Hills, MI: Minerva Press, 1995.

———. *Attention Deficit Disorder in Teenagers.* Bloomfield Hills, MI: Minerva Press, 1995.

———. *Attention Deficit Disorder: What Is It?* Bloomfield Hills, MI: Minerva Press, 1995.

Silver, Larry. *The Misunderstood Child: A Guide for Parents of Learning Disabled Children.* New York: McGraw-Hill, 1992.

———. *Dr. Larry Silver's Advice to Parents on Attention Deficit Hyperactivity Disorder.* Washington, D.C.: American Psychiatric Press, 1993.

Weiss, Gabrielle, and Lily Hechtman. *Hyperactive Children Grown Up: ADHD in Children, Adolescents and Adults,* 2nd ed. New York: Guilford Press, 1993.

Wender, Paul H. *The Hyperactive Child, Adolescent, and Adult: Attention Deficit Disorder Through the Lifespan.* New York: Oxford University Press, 1987.

Wodrich, D. *Attention Deficit Hyperactivity Disorder.* Baltimore: Paul H. Brooks, 1994.

RESOURCES

Children and Adults with Attention Deficit Disorder (CHADD)
8181 Professional Place, Suite 201
Landover, MD 20785
(301) 306-7070
Fax: (301) 306-7090

The Council for Exceptional Children
1920 Association Drive
Reston, VA 22091
(703) 620-3660
Fax: (703) 264-9494

Learning Disabilities Association
4156 Library Road
Pittsburgh, PA 15234
(412) 341-1515
Fax: (412) 344-0224

The National Attention Deficit Disorder Association
(ADDA)
9930 Johnnycake Ridge Road, Suite 3E
Mentor, OH 44060
(440) 350-9595

Tourette Syndrome Association (TSA)
42–40 Bell Boulevard, Suite 205
Bayside, NY 11361-2820
(718) 224-2999

Websites

**Children and Adults with Attention Deficit Disorders
(CHADD)**
  http://www.chadd.org/

Attention Deficit Disorders WWW Archive
  http://homepage.seas.upenn.edu/~mengwong/add/

National Attention Deficit Disorder Association
  http://www.add.org/

GLOSSARY

Adderall—a long-acting stimulant medication that is one of the newest stimulants on the market.

ADHD/ADD—common abbreviations for attention deficit disorder. ADD refers to attention deficit disorder, and ADHD to attention deficit hyperactivity disorder.

Aggression—a hostile or angry action that may result in harm to another person.

Antidepressant—a type of medication that slows the action of certain areas of the brain, reducing the symptoms of ADHD. Examples include Tofranil and Prozac.

Anxiety disorder—a condition characterized by severe nervousness or worrying. It is sometimes a comorbidity of ADHD.

Behavioral contract—a negotiated agreement between a parent and a child stipulating the behavior desired of the child and the resulting behavior (usually of a reinforcing nature) of the parent.

Bone marrow suppression—a rare side effect of Ritalin and other medications in which the body is unable to produce blood cells. This results in severe anemia and an inability to fight infections.

Brain stem—the deepest and most primitive section of the brain; it controls our basic functions.

Bupropion—an antidepressant medication that can be useful in the treatment of ADHD. Its brand name is Wellbutrin.

CAT scan—a computerized X ray that allows detailed examination of the body. It has been advocated by some experts to diagnose ADHD. Its name is an acronym for computerized axial tomography.

Catapres—the brand name of clonidine, a high blood pressure medication that can be useful in the treatment of ADHD.

Cerebellum—the section of the brain that controls complex movements and coordination.

Cerebral cortex—the most highly developed section of the brain. It controls all our thoughts, feelings, memories, sensations, and movements. The cortex is divided into two large sections called hemispheres, and each hemisphere is divided into sections called lobes.

Children and Adults with Attention Deficit Disorders (CHADD)—a national nonprofit group of parents, teachers, and professionals who are dedicated to helping kids and adults with ADHD. CHADD has many local chapters throughout the country.

Clonidine—a high blood pressure medication that can be useful in the treatment of ADHD. Its brand name is Catapres.

Cognitive behavioral therapy—a form of psychotherapy that combines the learning theories associated with behavioral therapy and the focus on faulty cognitions (thoughts and beliefs) of rational emotive therapy.

Comorbidity—a condition that occurs along with or is related to another condition. An example is the common coexistence of depression and ADHD.

Conners' Parent and Teacher Rating Scales— questionnaires commonly used to assess whether a child has ADHD or how well an ADHD child is responding to treatment.

Continuous Performance Test (CPT)—a computerized test used in ADHD evaluations to determine the subject's vigilance and sustained attention. Two of the best known such tests are the Gordon Diagnostic System and the Test of Variables of Attention (TOVA).

Corpus callosum—a thick band of nerves that connects the two sides of the brain.

Cylert—the brand name of pemoline, a long-acting stimulant medication used to treat ADHD.

Depression—a disorder characterized by a variety of symptoms, including an inability to focus, withdrawal, and sleep problems. It is a frequent comorbidity of ADHD.

Desipramine—an antidepressant medication that can be useful in the treatment of ADHD. Its brand name is Norpramin.

Dexedrine—the brand name of dextroamphetamine, a short-acting stimulant medication used to treat ADHD.

Dextroamphetamine—a short-acting stimulant medication used to treat ADHD. Its brand name is Dexedrine.

Distractibility—one of the predominant symptoms of attention deficit disorder. It is a trait whereby an outside stimulus interferes with or changes an individual's ability to focus or concentrate.

Deoxyribonucleic acid (DNA)—a large molecule found in every cell. It carries all the genetic information (or blueprints) for the body.

Dopamine—a chemical that the brain uses to communicate between two nerves. Also known as a neurotransmitter.

Diagnostic and Statistical Manual of Mental Disorders (DSM)—the bible for most mental health practioners. Published by the American Psychiatric Association, it is now in its fourth edition. It gives official diagnoses, assists in distinguishing between mental disorders, and gives statistical information on the prevalence of disorders. The current edition (*DSM-IV*), published in 1994, refers to attention deficit disorder as attention deficit hyperactivity disorder.

Education team—a group of school professionals assigned to handle special needs cases such as children with ADHD.

Electroencephalography (EEG)—a test that measures the brain's electrical activity. It is performed by attaching wires to a person's head and recording the brain waves. It is often used to diagnose seizures.

Epilepsy—a disorder in which a person suffers recurrent attacks of seizures.

Flattening—a rare side effect of several ADHD medications in which the child's personality and emotions become dulled or sluggish. It can often be reversed by adjusting the dosage of the drug or by switching to a different medication.

Fluoxetine—an antidepressant medication that can be useful in the treatment of ADHD. The brand name is Prozac.

Frontal lobe—the section of the brain that filters the vast amounts of information from the senses. This is the section that is most often dysfunctional in ADHD.

Gene—a portion of the DNA molecule that carries the code for a particular disease or characteristic.

Generic prescription drug—a drug sold as a chemically equivalent product by someone other than the original or established manufacturer.

Growth suppression—a questionable side effect associated with Ritalin in which there is a slowing of the growth process.

Haldol—the brand name of haloperidol, a tranquilizer used in the treatment of tics that can also be useful in the treatment of ADHD.

Haloperidol—a tranquilizer used in the treatment of tics that can also be useful in the treatment of ADHD. Its brand name is Haldol.

Home schooling—a legally recognized alternative to public and private schooling in which parents elect to teach the child at home.

Hyperactivity—one of several predominant symptoms of ADHD. Hyperactivity is an excessive amount of activity and energy. When it is present, the disorder is called ADHD or attention deficit hyperactivity disorder.

Imipramine—an antidepressant medication that can be useful in the treatment of ADHD. The brand name is Tofranil.

Impulsivity—one of several predominant symptoms of ADHD. Impulsivity refers to an individual's quick and often unthinking responses to a stimulus.

Learning disability—is a specific problem that impairs a person's ability to learn, like dyslexia or problems perceiving spatial relationships.

Manic-depressive disorder—a psychiatric condition characterized by episodes of extreme sadness followed by excessive euphoria and activity.

Methylphenidate—a short-acting stimulant medication used to treat ADHD. Its brand name is Ritalin.

Minimal brain dysfunction—an outdated name for ADHD.

Magnetic resonance imaging (MRI)—a sophisticated, computerized imaging scan that images the brain. It has been used to diagnose ADHD.

Multimodal treatment—therapy that involves several modes or methods. For instance, the treatment of ADHD includes medication, psychotherapy, classroom management, and parent training.

Neurological examination—an evaluation of a person's reflexes, balance, coordination, and strength. An abnormality in any of these areas does not indicate ADHD, but a neurological exam can help rule out other disorders.

Neuron—brain cells that conduct signals around the brain and body like tiny wires. The human brain is made up of more than 100 billion neurons.

Neurotransmitter—a chemical that allows two neurons to communicate across a synaptic space. Examples include dopamine, norepinephrine, epinephrine, and serotonin.

Norepinephrine—a chemical that the brain uses to communicate between two nerves. Also known as a neurotransmitter.

Norpramin—the brand name of desipramine, an antidepressant medication that can be useful in the treatment of ADHD.

Occipital lobe—the section of the brain that processes all visual information.

Oppositional defiant disorder (ODD)—a disorder characterized by rebellious or disobedient behavior and excessive anger. Often a comorbidity or result of ADHD.

Parietal lobe—the section of the brain that controls sensation and movement.

Pemoline—a long-acting stimulant medication used to treat ADHD. Its brand name is Cylert.

Petit mal seizure—a type of seizure in which the person temporarily lapses into a trancelike state lasting less than a minute.

Positron-emission tomography (PET)—a sophisticated brain scan that measures the metabolic activity of the brain. It has been used to diagnose ADHD.

Placebo—an inactive medication or "sugar pill" often used in controlled experiments. It is given to make a patient in a study think he or she is receiving a medication.

Post-traumatic stress disorder—a condition characterized by extreme anxiety following a severe stress (like a car accident or a tornado). The symptoms include nightmares, depression, and difficulty concentrating. These symptoms can take years to become evident.

Prozac—the brand name of fluoxetine, an antidepressant medication that can be useful in the treatment of ADHD.

Rating scale—a questionnaire used to assess whether a child has ADHD or how well he is responding to treatment. It is given to both teachers and parents to fill out, and then the responses are compared with responses to prior questionnaires or standard values. Commonly used rating scales include the Conners' Teacher Rating Scale, the Conners' Parent Rating Scale—Revised, the Home Situations Questionnaire—Revised, and the Child Behavior Checklist—Parent Form.

Rebound—a worsening of the symptoms of ADHD after the medication has worn off.

Ritalin—the brand name of methylphenidate, a short-acting stimulant medication used to treat ADHD.

Ritalin roller coaster—the up-and-down effect that Ritalin can have on a few children's emotions. It can often be reversed by adjusting the dosage of Ritalin or switching to a different medication.

Seizure—a sudden, uncontrollable muscular contraction caused by abnormal electrical discharges from the brain. Also called *convulsion*.

Self-concept—the combined feelings, ideas, and beliefs that a person has about his identity.

Self-esteem—the mental image a person has of herself, and her sense of value as a person. It is often affected in ADHD children who are not treated.

Serotonin—a chemical that the brain uses to communicate between two nerves. Also known as a neurotransmitter.

Short attention span—one of the predominant symptoms of ADHD. Attention span is the length of time an activity is pursued without interruption.

Social skills—a person's ability to communicate and solve interpersonal problems. Individuals with ADHD often have difficulties with social skills.

Single photon emission computer tomography (SPECT)—a sophisticated computerized imaging scan that is used to study the brain. It has been used to diagnose ADHD.

Stimulant—a type of medication that activates certain areas of the brain, reducing the symptoms of ADHD. Examples include Ritalin and Cylert.

Substance abuse—the self-destructive use of illegal or legal drugs and/or alcohol.

Synapse—a connection or communication point between two neurons. Neurons communicate over a synapse by means of a neurotransmitter.

Temperament—the inborn, genetic, and enduring traits that determine how an individual responds to the world. Temperamental traits include activity level, attention span, persistence, adaptability to change, mood, sensitivity, and distractibility.

Temporal lobe—the section of the brain that processes all sounds and stores memories. Some of the symptoms of ADHD may be related to dysfunction in this section.

Tic—a repetitive and involuntary movement, often in the face or the extremities.

Time-out—a discipline technique that involves removing a child from a scene of intense action to a dull, nonstimulating place, often a special time-out place. It can be a chair in a hallway or facing a wall, or stair steps on which the child is to sit. Since it is a punishment, time-out should be used only to decrease more dangerous or serious behavior. Overuse of this or any other punishment will decrease its effectiveness, and the child will become immune to your use of it.

Tofranil—the brand name of imipramine, an antidepressant medication that can be useful in the treatment of ADHD.

Tourette's syndrome—a condition characterized by uncontrollable movements or tics, often of the face. It is thought to be closely related to ADHD.

Wellbutrin—the brand name of bupropion, an antidepressant medication that can be useful in the treatment of ADHD.

Zombie/zombie effect—a reported side effect of Ritalin, in which a parent perceives a child as acting as if he or she is in a stupor or is less active.

INDEX

ABOUT THE AUTHORS

JAMES SHAYA, M.D., F.A.A.P. is a pediatrician with the Mercy Medical Group in Clarkston, Michigan, who works with ADHD children and their parents. He writes a weekly column for *The Oakland Press* in Oakland County, Michigan. Dr. Shaya is a Fellow of the American Academy of Pediatrics and a Diplomat of the American Board of Pediatrics.

JAMES WINDELL, M.A. is a psychologist with the Oakland (Michigan) County Juvenile Court, who in his private practice works with many adolescents affected by ADHD. He is the author of *Discipline: A Sourcebook of 50 Failsafe Techniques for Parents* (Collier), *8 Weeks to a Well-Behaved Child* (Macmillan) and *Children Who Say No When You Want Them to Say Yes* (Macmillan).

HOLLY SHREVE GILBERT is a writer, former newspaper editor at *The Oakland Press*, and instructor of journalism at Oakland University in Rochester, MI.

Create Your Own Medical Library with
☑ Bantam Medical Reference Books

The Bantam Medical Dictionary
by the editors of Market House Books

Offering the latest authoritative definitions in simple language, this exhaustive reference covers anatomy, physiology, all the major medical and surgical specialties from cardiology to tropical medicine. It also discusses fields such as biochemistry, nutrition, pharmacology, psychology, psychiatry, and dentistry.

❏ 28498-3 $6.99/$8.99 in Canada

The Pill Book
8th edition

More than 1,500 drugs in this revised edition--25 newly approved

Profiles of the 1,500 most commonly prescribed drugs in the United States: generic and brand names, dosages, side effects, adverse reactions, and warnings. Includes 32 pages of actual-size color photographs of prescription pills, as well as information on drugs with food, sex, pregnancy, alcohol, children, and the elderly.

❏ 57971-1 $6.99/$8.99 in Canada

Ask for these books at your local bookstore or use this page to order.

Please send me the books I have checked above. I am enclosing $_____ (add $2.50 to cover postage and handling). Send check or money order, no cash or C.O.D.'s, please.

Name _____

Address _____

City/State/Zip _____

Send order to: Bantam Books, Dept. HN 13, 2451 S. Wolf Rd., Des Plaines, IL 60018
Allow four to six weeks for delivery.

Prices and availability subject to change without notice.   HN 13 12/96